Obsessive Compulsive Disorder

All You Want to Know about OCD for
People Living with OCD, Carers, and
Clinicians

Lynne M. Drummond
South West London and St George's Mental Health NHS Trust

with

Laura J. Edwards

CAMBRIDGE
UNIVERSITY PRESS

CAMBRIDGE
UNIVERSITY PRESS

University Printing House, Cambridge CB2 8BS, United Kingdom

One Liberty Plaza, 20th Floor, New York, NY 10006, USA

477 Williamstown Road, Port Melbourne, VIC 3207, Australia

314–321, 3rd Floor, Plot 3, Splendor Forum, Jasola District Centre, New Delhi – 110025, India

79 Anson Road, #06-04/06, Singapore 079906

Cambridge University Press is part of the University of Cambridge.

It furthers the University's mission by disseminating knowledge in the pursuit of education, learning, and research at the highest international levels of excellence.

www.cambridge.org
Information on this title: www.cambridge.org/9781911623755
DOI: 10.1017/9781911623335

First published 2018
Reprinted 2018

Printed and bound in Great Britain by Clays Ltd, Elcograf S.p.A.

A catalogue record for this publication is available from the British Library.

Library of Congress Cataloging-in-Publication Data
Names: Drummond, Lynne M., author.
Title: Obsessive compulsive disorder : all you want to know about OCD for people living with OCD, carers, and clinicians / Lynne M. Drummond, St. George's Hospital Medical School, University of London with Laura J. Edwards.
Description: New York, NY : Cambridge University Press, 2018.
Identifiers: LCCN 2018009837 | ISBN 9781911623755 (paperback)
Subjects: LCSH: Obsessive-compulsive disorder. | Obsessive-compulsive disorder—Treatment. | Obsessive-compulsive disorder—Research. | BISAC: MEDICAL / Mental Health.
Classification: LCC RC533 .D78 2018 | DDC 616.85/227—dc23 LC record available at https://lccn.loc.gov/2018009837

ISBN 978-1-911-62375-5 Paperback

Obsessive Compulsive Disorder

All You Want to Know about OCD for People Living with OCD, Carers, and Clinicians

Contents

Contents

Preface

This book arose out of my experience, dating back to the 1980s, with people living with obsessive compulsive disorder (OCD) and their families. When I was developing my interest in this area, few people had heard of OCD, and those who had were often confused about what it was. Today there appears, at first sight, to be much greater awareness. However, a higher profile in the media has also led to a frequent underestimation about how damaging and severe OCD can be. People now frequently quip that they are 'a bit OCD', not understanding that in its severe forms, OCD destroys relationships and families and can lead to the early demise of the individual. OCD does not just comprise being fussy or preferring an orderly life; it is also a serious, life-restricting psychological disorder which requires help and treatment. Fortunately, there are now good and effective treatments which can alter the prognosis of OCD and lead to people living happy, fulfilled lives with minimal inconvenience from OCD symptoms. Despite this, there is still confusion regarding the evidenced-based treatments and how to ensure that people receive the appropriate help and care they need. I hope this book will help bridge the gap.

This book first describes OCD and how it can impact families. Next, it provides a full discussion concerning tried and tested treatments. The book then examines more 'experimental' and unusual treatments for the handful of individuals who do not gain benefit from standard treatments.

Throughout the book, I illustrate the discussion using the stories of patients I have met throughout the years. None of these stories is based on any one individual; rather, the stories are accumulations of many hundreds of individuals. Any similarity to any one individual is purely accidental and does not represent that individual in any way. I have tried to give practical and realistic advice to people living with OCD, their families, and healthcare professionals. I hope you find the book useful, informative, and empowering.

Chapter

1

What Is OCD and Is It Really a Problem?

This chapter will examine a brief overview of obsessive compulsive disorder (OCD) and its defining features. Public perception of OCD over time will then be appraised, from the low awareness that existed throughout much of the early twentieth century to the present, when it is almost fashionable to claim that an individual is 'a little bit OCD'.

The chapter will then examine what distinguishes 'normal' obsessions and compulsions from those that are detrimental to the individual and their functioning. Finally, the chapter explores how obsessions and compulsions may have evolved and how they may give the individual a biological advantage.

What Is OCD?

Obsessive compulsive disorder is one of the most overlooked and frequently misdiagnosed conditions. People often talk about a friend or family member being 'obsessed' by a particular football team, a hobby, or a girlfriend/boyfriend. In addition, someone who is organised, works hard, and is generally neat and tidy may describe him- or herself or be described by others as 'slightly OCD'. The behaviours in these cases are often very different from the extreme symptoms with which many patients with OCD suffer.

A person with OCD has two major symptoms: obsessions and compulsions. Obsessions are troublesome and persistent thoughts or impulses which appear in a person's mind and result in anxiety, horror, or disgust. Because these thoughts are often so unpleasant, the person will resist the thoughts and try to ignore them or force them away. Unfortunately, trying to push the thoughts away often results in them recurring more frequently. These obsessive and intrusive thoughts are generally the worst thoughts that the individual can imagine. For example, a religious person may have blasphemous thoughts; a gentle and loving parent may have images of harming their child; or a person with high moral standards may have worries that they have been acting in an inappropriate sexual way towards another, despite evidence to the contrary.

Obsessive thoughts cause the person to be very anxious and uncomfortable. Normally when a person is frightened, they will attempt to escape from the

1

situation. In the case of anxiety-provoking thoughts, it is impossible to escape from them; as a result, a number of compulsions are developed. Compulsions are thoughts or behaviours which are designed to reduce or prevent the harm of the obsessive thought. However, either they are not realistically linked with the obsession or they are clearly excessive. Compulsions tend to reduce anxiety, and because high anxiety is unpleasant, the decrease in anxiety following the performance of a compulsion is rather like a reward to the individual. If you reward any behaviour, you increase the chances of it happening in similar circumstances in the future. This means that by causing a reduction in anxiety, the tendency to perform compulsions becomes stronger the more they are repeated. In addition, compulsions will only slightly reduce anxiety over a short space of time, and so individuals will repeat the compulsive behaviours until they feel 'right' or until another thought distracts them.

Case Study 1.1

Anne is a 30-year-old married woman who used to work as a teaching assistant. She has always been a conscientious and capable woman, and she worked hard at her job. After giving birth to her daughter Lily at age 28 years, Anne became increasingly worried that she might 'poison' Lily with dirt and germs, which would result in Lily becoming ill or dying. Most mothers worry about cleanliness around a baby, but in Anne's case, this quickly got out of control. She was not content with using sterilising fluid on Lily's utensils; rather, she would repeat the action many times. In addition, she began to wash her hands increasingly until she was eventually washing them more than 100 times a day. Once Lily was mobile and walking around, Anne began to clean every area where Lily might play and then began to prevent Lily from playing outside. Anne realises that her concerns are excessive, but due to her overwhelming anxiety, she is unable to ignore her thoughts and she feels the urge to 'play safe' by performing her compulsive rituals.

In Anne's situation, her compulsions are linked to her desire to be a good mother, but her worries and her 'decontamination' compulsions are excessive and beyond normal cleanliness. This overconcern about Lily is actually restricting Lily's ability to learn and play and to explore the world.

Case Study 1.2

Amy is a 25-year-old woman who fears that she might cause a catastrophic fire if she does not ensure she has turned off all electrical appliances and the gas cooker. After using appliances, she repeatedly checks that they are switched off, returning up to 50 times. In the past two years, she has tried to avoid using all electrical or gas appliances and asks her mother, with whom she lives, to use these for her. If she does have to use an appliance, she will repeatedly ask her mother for reassurance that she has not caused a fire. Her mother will reassure her, but a few minutes later, Amy will ask again, and this can continue for many hours until Amy has a new worry. If Amy's mother refuses to answer the questions, Amy becomes extremely tearful and upset, and her mother will then relent and give her the reassurance.

Amy's story shows that compulsions can sometimes take the form of reassurance seeking. Just like checking, counting, and decontamination compulsive rituals, these activities can also slightly reduce anxiety. Because high anxiety is unpleasant, this reduction in anxiety is similar to a reward. If any behaviour is 'rewarded', the chance that it will reoccur in similar circumstances increases. This means that the compulsions increase the more they are repeated. By providing reassurance, Amy's mother is trying to help her daughter and alleviate her distress but is accidentally making the situation worse.

Case Study 1.3

Jim is a 35-year-old man who has always wanted to ensure that he does the 'right' thing, and he prides himself on holding high moral standards. He was popular in school and left school having passed his exams. There were no obvious signs of OCD during his early life, and he had close friends, although he had never formed a lasting sexual relationship. Jim has worked as a security guard since leaving school, and he managed well until four years ago. At that time, Jim read about some high-profile celebrities who had been involved in child sexual abuse. Jim was appalled and shocked by these revelations and was clear that he believed such behaviour was 'evil'. However, he began to check that he himself had not inadvertently sexually assaulted a child. These concerns have led him to completely avoid any place where there may be children. Parks, roads with schools or nurseries, and even buses at peak times before and after school have become 'out of bounds' for Jim. If he does unexpectedly see a child, he will tightly squeeze his hands into fists, cross his arms across his body, and stand totally still until they leave. This behaviour is an attempt to ensure that he does not 'lurch at the child and assault them'. Once they have passed, he still doubts himself and repeatedly taps his right foot on the ground in multiples of 20 until he feels sure he remained motionless on the spot when the child went past. Occasionally, he has been stuck in this position for 15–20 minutes after seeing a child. Jim realises that this behaviour is unconnected with his fears, and he understands that he has not attacked a child. Nonetheless, the fear is so great that he feels compelled to perform the compulsive foot tapping. Occasionally, he has placed himself in danger as a result of this behaviour by becoming 'stuck' in the middle of busy roads. The OCD has also resulted in Jim having to stop working due to his attempt to avoid children.

In the case of Jim, it is clear that the obsessional thoughts are completely abhorrent to him, and he is the opposite of someone who would enjoy sexually abusing children because he finds the thought so awful. His behaviours to avoid this are excessive and, in the case of the foot-tapping compulsion, are not actually connected with the obsessive fear. In addition, Jim's story demonstrates his increasing avoidance and restriction of daily activities due to OCD.

People with OCD tend to progressively avoid objects or situations which provoke the obsessive thoughts. Due to this avoidance, their lives can become increasingly more restricted and limited. This is demonstrated in the previous case studies. Anne increasingly handed over some of her child care to either her mother or her husband as her fears progressed. Amy increasingly stopped using electrical appliances and demanded her mother cook and switch off appliances for her. Jim's life became increasingly restricted as he avoided all areas where children and young people might be present.

But We All Have Some OCD, Don't We?

Most of us experience some kind of obsessions and compulsions. Many people will, for example, throw salt over their left shoulder in response to spilling salt, due to a European belief that this will scare the devil away. Others will salute or cross their fingers if they see a solitary magpie, which has traditionally been linked with sorrow. These behaviours are similar to obsessions and compulsions, but they tend not to be repetitive and also do not cause extreme distress or interfere with a person's ability to perform normal activities of daily living.

Obsessive thoughts have been experienced by many of us when standing on the top of a high building or on the platform as a train is about to arrive and we suddenly have the thought or urge that we may throw ourselves over the side. This thought is unpleasant, and we may take a step back. Similarly, most of us have experienced sudden violent, blasphemous, or inappropriate sexual thoughts. Generally, we will have these thoughts and then dismiss them as being 'stupid' or 'inappropriate' and forget about them. It appears that most people with OCD are not able to do this. Many will have a thought and find it so overwhelmingly unpleasant or worrying that they try very hard to never have that thought again. Of course, once you try *not* to have a thought, the thought will continue happening as you keep it in your mind.

The fact that all of us experience some obsessions and may perform some compulsions shows that along with many other psychological and mental disturbances, OCD is on a spectrum. Although it is not difficult to recognise that people who are spending almost all their time preoccupied by their obsessive fears and compulsive rituals have a problem, people often ask the question, 'When is OCD a problem that needs help?' The answer to this question depends on the individual. OCD traits seem to be at least partially genetically inherited. Some of the traits that many OCD patients have – being conscientious, meticulous, and punctual – are clearly an advantage in life. There is no mystery in the fact that many sufferers of OCD have been highly successful as doctors, nurses, accountants, lawyers, secretaries, and journalists and in other professions which require high attention to detail and the ability to concentrate well for hours on end. It is easy to see that there may be a biological advantage to humans to have some obsessive traits. Avoidance of excrement and disgust are traits which humans share with many other animals. From the Stone Age (or even earlier), an individual who avoided faeces would clearly have a biological advantage over one who did not. Similarly, someone who was persistent and meticulous would also often have an advantage in survival terms over someone who was not. However, it is when these traits become overwhelming and take over every other aspect of the individual's life that the issue becomes a problem.

Case Study 1.4

Geoff is a 25-year-old man whose parents were both doctors; his mother worked as a general practitioner, and his father was an orthopaedic surgeon. The family has three children. The eldest child, George, is a solicitor working in a successful law firm. Molly, the middle child, is an academic historian working at a prestigious university. Geoff was similarly a high-achieving scholar in the early years of his schooling but began to fail to achieve predicted grades once he reached the age of 13. His parents were concerned at the time, and Geoff was seen by a child psychologist. Not wishing to admit to the problems he was experiencing, Geoff denied any difficulties despite the evidence to the contrary. The family was offered family therapy, and Geoff's teachers believed he was experiencing 'adolescent rebellion'. In fact, Geoff had become concerned that he had to get everything perfect and correct or else he would feel a failure. He was not able to describe what 'being a failure' may constitute except that it was a 'terrible, bad thing' and that his family and friends 'would not respect' him. Occasionally, he admits that he believes that not being perfect would lead to him being abandoned by everyone he loves. He finds this thought so frightening that he becomes paralysed with fear, checking that everything he does is performed 100 per cent correctly. For example, he was meticulous at school with his handwriting and, consequently, he was predicted to easily pass his school examinations with the highest grades. However, he failed or gained borderline grades due to his meticulous attention to detail, resulting in his inability to complete the examinations within the allotted time.

As the years passed and his fear of failure continued, his symptoms worsened. Currently, he is unable to perform any activity without extreme distress. Washing and bathing take up to eight hours as he tries to ensure that he washes his body perfectly. Consequently, he has given up his daily bath and now showers when he believes he 'has the time'. This has meant that he has not bathed for more than six months. Similarly, his fingernails and toenails are long and curled because he cannot bear to make a mistake when trimming them. His hair is matted and unkempt, as otherwise he would worry that the barber had not cut his hair perfectly straight. Wearing a long straggly beard because he is unable to attempt shaving, he makes a sharp contrast with his pristine and well-groomed parents and siblings.

Summary

The history of Geoff shows that his high-achieving and slightly perfectionist family members all managed to succeed in life in spite of, or maybe because of, these characteristics. Geoff, on the other hand, became so caught up in perfectionism that it has impaired his ability to function in activities of daily living and his ability to work. It is clear to everyone that Geoff's fear of performing an action imperfectly means that he is far from perfect – the situation he is fearful of! This 'all-or-nothing' or 'black-and-white' thinking is frequently observed in people with a desire to achieve perfection. They seem unable to compromise and are happier to accept the state of total failure rather than try to perform an action and risk not doing it perfectly. In other words, they seem unable to find the 'happy medium' and be 'good enough' rather than perfect. Realistically, perfection is not a normal human state, and anyone who seeks to achieve it is likely to fall short to some degree. It is more realistic to try to arrive at a happy compromise of being 'fit for purpose'!

Key Points

- Obsessive compulsive disorder (OCD) consists of obsessions and compulsions.
- Obsessions are thoughts, ideas, images, or impulses which are deeply unpleasant and result in increased anxiety or distress.
- Compulsions are thoughts or actions which are designed to reduce or prevent the effect of the obsession. However, either they are not realistically related to obsessive fear or they are clearly excessive. Many patients seek repeated reassurance from their friends, family, or others as a form of compulsive behaviour.
- Avoidance is also frequently seen in people with OCD. People will often progressively avoid objects and situations which may provoke the OCD thoughts. The consequence of this avoidance is that the individual may live an increasingly restricted life and may end up unable to work or socially very isolated.
- The symptoms of both obsessions and compulsions are found in the general population amongst people who do not necessarily suffer from OCD. The difference between obsessions and compulsions in OCD and these more 'normal' obsessions and compulsions is that they do not take over the person's life nor do they restrict the person's ability to achieve their life aims.

Chapter 2

Who Gets OCD and How Would Anyone Know If They Had It?

We will now examine who can develop OCD and why this might happen. We will look at population data on OCD. The role of inheritance, genetics, and possible environmental factors will be discussed, as well as the idea of developing resilience. Next, we will explore OCD throughout the life cycle. OCD is a common disorder in childhood and seems to have some differences compared to adult-onset OCD. Following a discussion of OCD in childhood or early adult life, we will look at how the pattern changes throughout the years and into middle and old age.

This chapter will also examine how culture may have an effect on the presentation of OCD. For example, all religions involve ritual and symbolic behaviours which have some similarities to OCD but generally do not take over a person's life. When OCD features religious ideas, other members of the same religion can often distinguish that the person with OCD is taking this to an extreme.

Who Gets OCD?

In Chapter 1, we briefly discussed the role that inheritance may play in developing OCD and how some obsessive traits may be helpful in developing a successful life path. In the case of OCD, the obsessions and compulsions become overwhelming and interfere with the person's life objectives, aims, and ambitions. OCD can affect people of any gender and of any social class, race, nationality, or religion.

Many years ago, OCD was thought to be a rare condition. Large population studies performed in the 1980s showed that this was untrue and that 2 or 3 per cent of the population suffer from OCD during their lifetime [1]. Of course, estimating the prevalence of OCD is not an easy task. Many people with OCD are ashamed and embarrassed by their condition and will go to great lengths to try to hide it rather than admit to problems. It has been found that some people with OCD may resist seeking help for decades. In addition, population studies may run the risk of including people with mild obsessions and compulsions which do not interfere with their lives, and this may falsely increase the numbers. Generally, it seems that the figure of 2 or 3 per cent of the population is accurate for most societies.

Population studies generally suggest that women with OCD outnumber men with OCD by a ratio of 1.5:1. The interesting twist in this fact is that with regard to hospital, clinic, and professional referrals, more men than women are referred for help. This may be because men tend to have more severe conditions compared to women. Alternatively, it might be that men's absences from work are more likely to be noticed than women's absences. Women more frequently have washing compulsions and avoidance, whereas men more frequently have checking compulsions or complex thought compulsions. Of course, these trends, based on large populations of people with OCD, do not mean that a woman cannot have the most profound OCD with thought compulsions or that a man cannot have washing rituals; they simply demonstrate overall trends in the population.

The average age of onset of OCD is approximately 20 years. However, there does appear to be a peak of development of OCD around or just before puberty and then a much larger peak of onset in early adult life. Men are more likely to report that their OCD started in their early teens, whereas women more commonly have an onset in their early 20s. These figures are averages, and OCD does occur at extremely young ages and also at older ages. It is quite rare for OCD to develop without any earlier symptoms after the age of 40 years, and in such cases, further tests are usually advisable to ensure there are no other complications.

Until recently, it was thought to be unusual for children to suffer from OCD. Now it is known that OCD is, in fact, one of the most common mental disorders in childhood and may affect up to 5 per cent of children and adolescents. The clinical presentation in childhood is similar to that seen in adults. Again, boys tend to develop the condition earlier than do girls. The prognosis for OCD in childhood is generally better than that for adults.

If Someone in My Family Has OCD, Does That Mean I Will Get It?

The issue of genetics and psychological problems and mental illness is a complex one. Most conditions are not caused by a single gene but, rather, are 'multifactorial'. In other words, the characteristics may run in families, but not everyone in a family will suffer from the condition. The same is true for OCD. What also appears to be true is that even if an individual inherits a very strong chance of suffering from OCD, it is not guaranteed that he or she will develop the condition. Increasingly, research seems to show that the way in which genes express themselves can be modified by external events. Some people, even within the same family, appear more prone than others to developing problems. This resilience seems likely to be partly inherited and partly a result of upbringing and early life experience. In the past, parents often took responsibility for causing their offspring's psychological problems due to poor parenting. This is clearly unfair and not the case. Parents share some of their genes with their offspring, and so parenting styles are partly influenced by their own genetic makeup and personality. Second, although it appears likely that a warm, loving family environment may provide the offspring with somewhat greater resilience, this can never be absolute. People from the very best families who have received an abundance of warmth, love, and the best parenting can still develop psychological problems. The genes are still the main deciding factor.

Not even the happiest and most loving family experience can completely prevent OCD from occurring in some individuals. The pattern of age of onset for OCD reflects this idea. Most adult patients with OCD develop it in early adult life and often in association with a major negative life event. In these cases, it may be reasonable to assume that the individual had a high genetic susceptibility to OCD and that, due to the individual's resilience, it took a major life event for OCD to be manifest; that the individual had moderate genetic susceptibility to OCD and poor resilience; or that the individual had a low susceptibility to OCD, and an extremely traumatic life event coupled with low resilience resulted in OCD. Therefore, it can be seen that factors which may determine whether or not an individual develops OCD include their genetic makeup, resilience (which is likely to be due to both genetics and early life nurturing), and the scale and impact of the negative life event.

A smaller but still significant number of adults with OCD develop it before puberty. These individuals are slightly more likely to be male rather than female. It has also been noted that they may have some specific neurological signs which do not interfere with normal functioning but may suggest high genetic loading for OCD.

What Will Happen If You Do Develop OCD?

Many children who develop OCD go on to recover; OCD is one of the most common psychological problems seen in childhood. Most children will experience a phase of OCD-like behaviours which will resolve in time. Other children go on to develop OCD, but the prognosis is extremely good. Apart from the small group of individuals who go on to develop long-standing OCD into adulthood, most children who are treated for OCD respond well and recover completely. Treatment for childhood OCD is mostly psychological, but short-term drug use can also be helpful for some children.

The course that OCD takes when untreated is variable. Some people may have occasional, discrete episodes interspersed with periods during which they are symptom-free. These episodes are often precipitated by stress surrounding a major life event, such as bereavement, illness, pregnancy, or loss of a job. Some people with apparent very late-onset OCD may develop this after retirement, but careful examination of the life history can show that there may have been previous short-lived episodes of OCD or strong OCD tendencies which were controlled by the discipline of working. Other people develop OCD and it remains at a similar level for many years until successfully treated. Another group of people may have OCD which is consistently present but which waxes and wanes throughout the years; sometimes these variations are related to life circumstances at the time, and sometimes they are apparently unrelated. Finally, a small group develops OCD which becomes increasingly restrictive over the years. The content of the obsessions in all types of OCD may change throughout the years, or in some cases it will remain consistent.

Because many people with OCD often do not seek help for years or even decades, fewer of them are married or in cohabiting relationships than would be expected based on their age. Many people with OCD live alone, and a significant number live with their parents. OCD can be a huge burden on families because they feel the need to comply with the OCD 'rules' of their family member. The prime consideration must always be the well-being of any children. OCD in a parent can lead to a restricted life for any children present. Everyone involved with a person with OCD needs to ensure that children are free to have as happy and carefree lives as possible and are able to play normally inside and outside the home and interact with their peers. Some people with OCD live with aging parents, who are called on to perform functions to help their children at an age when they would normally be autonomous.

Case Study 2.1

Fred is a 45-year-old man who has suffered from OCD with fear of contamination for 25 years. He lives with his 85-year-old parents. Due to his OCD, Fred believes he is unable to shower himself because he thinks he may not do it 'sufficiently'. He insists that his parents shower him once a week. These showers must be performed according to Fred's strict OCD 'rules'. When his parents refuse to comply with these 'rules', Fred becomes angry and threatening.

Fred's story shows how the family, as well as the sufferer, can become completely enveloped in OCD. It is never acceptable for an individual to be coerced into performing OCD compulsive rituals for another person. Violence and threats cannot be tolerated. The problem is often that parents of the person with OCD may feel guilty about their son's or daughter's plight, wrongly thinking it is their 'fault'. Most parents do not like to see their offspring suffer and so will start to perform some of the compulsive rituals for them in the hope of easing the distress. Unfortunately, this help can escalate until the whole family is 'imprisoned' by the OCD. In addition, parents can unwittingly worsen the situation by delaying the time until people such as Fred seek help.

As well as fewer people with OCD being married or living with a partner, fewer are employed compared to the general population of the same age. Some people have OCD and work in jobs in which some minor OCD traits may appear to be an advantage. These traits can also frequently get out of control.

Case Study 2.2

Jenny, a 20-year-old student nurse, has recently become extremely concerned that she may cause an infection to spread to a patient in her current placement on an elderly ward. The hospital has strict policy guidance about staff hand washing and the use of protective gowns and gloves when handling bodily fluids. However, Jenny fears these do not go far enough. She insists on wearing a new pair of gloves for every activity, which is beyond the hospital guidance on infection. If she has to prepare a sterile trolley for a doctor to perform a blood test, she will take up to an hour to ensure it is clean and sterile. Rather than just cleaning the surface once, she will repeatedly clean the trolley until she believes it is 'just right'. Although at first the more senior staff believed Jenny would settle into the job and become less anxious, the charge nurse is now planning to fail her for this placement due to her slowness and overly meticulous behaviour.

Case Study 2.3

George is a 30-year-old architect. He is studious and hard-working and is generally appreciated by his boss. For the past ten years, George has been overly concerned that he may make an error which would result in either a catastrophic problem with a building he has been working on or lead to him losing his job. George arrives at work at 7:00 a.m. every morning, which is two hours before he is due at work. He rarely leaves work before 7:00 p.m., and even then he tends to take home files and work on his computer at home, checking and rechecking his calculations repeatedly. On weekends, he generally works 15–18 hours a day checking and rechecking his work. Due to these excessive hours, he often fails to eat or drink sufficiently and has found that he feels permanently exhausted and cannot sleep well at night. Despite working the extra hours, George has not yet been noted to have any difficulty by his work colleagues, who are unaware of the number of hours he is working.

These examples demonstrate how OCD can impact the working environment. In Jenny's case, she is too slow and careful to perform her job usefully. George is performing well and the amount of time he works is currently unknown by his superiors, but his excessive working hours are impacting his general health and well-being.

Is OCD New and Caused by Modern Society? What about Religion and Culture?

OCD is not a modern-day disease of the Western world; rather, there is evidence of its existence in historical figures as well as across all cultures. John Bunyan, the author of *Pilgrim's Progress*, was born in 1628, and it has been suggested that he may have suffered from OCD. In his spiritual autobiography, Bunyan, a strict Christian, describes blasphemous thoughts repeatedly entering his mind. He found these thoughts deeply abhorrent and repeatedly tried to distract himself or to 'put this right' by saying he did not mean these thoughts. A more modern example is that of the famous film producer, aviator, aircraft manufacturer, successful businessman, and playboy, Howard Hughes. He suffered from obsessions concerning his health and fear of death. Despite being a multimillionaire, he became increasingly concerned about his health and developed an extreme lifestyle. Ultimately, he lived the life of a recluse, living in a bare room with no clothes and eating and drinking at starvation levels. This self-neglect may have led to a hastening of his death at the age of 71 years.

OCD has been found in very different cultures throughout the world. There have been reports of OCD with similar characteristics and a similar prevalence amongst the Han population in China and the ultra-Orthodox Jewish population in Israel, as well as similar reports from Iran, India, and Western countries. The detailed content of the obsessions may vary from culture to culture – for example, it has been noted that the ultra-Orthodox Jewish person with OCD tends to have obsessions related to religious teachings – but the forms these obsessions take are indistinguishable throughout the world.

In the past, it was often argued that certain religious upbringings may lead to OCD. There is no evidence that this is true. There does seem to be a tendency for people with OCD to be attracted to more dogmatic branches of religions, in which there is a firm stance on what is 'right' and what is 'wrong', rather than more philosophical beliefs, in which there is less certainty. OCD is not, however, related to any specific religion; it has been reported in Christians, Muslims, Jews, Hindus, Buddhists, Confucians, and Taoists, as well as atheists and agnostics. It was once thought that the religions themselves may precipitate OCD. This was first reported in Italy, where a higher proportion of people with OCD were found in religious orders than in the outside population. However, it seems more likely that people with OCD were more attracted to the certainty and security of religious life rather than the religion itself being a causal factor. All religions have ritualistic and symbolic aspects which may resemble OCD. Some people with OCD believe that their religion requires them to carry out their OCD behaviours. Overall, it seems that whereas some people with OCD-like tendencies or even real OCD may be attracted to the stricter forms of religion, there is no evidence that any religion causes OCD. Religions with a more rigid 'black-and-white' approach to life seem to be particularly attractive to some people with OCD compared to religions with a more philosophical approach. People who practice religions and adhere to various religious rituals can generally be distinguished from people who perform their OCD compulsions to excess within their religions.

Case Study 2.4

Emma is a 45-year-old woman with a 30-year history of OCD. She worries that she may have harmed others and constantly checks to ensure this is not the case. In addition, she constantly asks for reassurance from family and friends that she has not committed the heinous act she is currently worrying about. If she reads about a terrible murder in the papers or sees a news bulletin describing such an event, she will check that she was not in the vicinity of the event and will then ask for repeated reassurance from her husband or others around her at the time that she did not commit the act. This is extremely difficult for her husband, who frequently is asked for reassurance for four or five hours at a time after he returns home from work. In the past, Emma frequently telephoned the police to 'confess' her guilt even though she based her confessions on only sketchy media reports about the crimes. She realises that she has no memory of the events but worries that she may have forgotten them. The police no longer pay any attention to her 'confessions', but on one occasion they took up the floorboards of her house because she was worried she may have murdered a man and hidden him there.

After many years of this behaviour, Emma resisted all offers of therapy but was befriended by a member of a local church. Emma began to attend the church, whose members believed in spiritual healing. Part of the spiritual healing involved not only other church members praying intensely for one to be healed but also public confession of one's sins. Emma became a regular attendee at these confession sessions, where she tended to dominate the proceedings with her current worries of crimes she may have committed. At first, the church was welcoming and tried to accommodate her. Soon, the members realised that she had a serious psychological problem. The minister approached her and suggested that she get referred for treatment. She was also told that although she was still most welcome to attend church, she was no longer welcome at the public confession sessions.

The story of Emma shows how a particular aspect of religion can become very attractive to someone with OCD. It also demonstrates that regular worshippers are able to identify a person who is taking the religion too far and needs help. People have been advised to seek help from a variety of religions when following religious rituals excessively. It may be useful for the therapist to work in conjunction with the local priest, mullah, minister, vicar, or rabbi with the consent of the person with OCD to ensure that treatment is truly in accordance with appropriate religious beliefs.

Key Points

- Although once thought to be a rare condition, OCD affects 2 or 3 per cent of the population and is therefore a very common disorder.
- Both men and women can be affected by OCD, and overall the gender ratio is approximately equal.
- Most people develop OCD in early adult life and often, but not always, following a negative life event.
- A smaller but significant number of adults with OCD developed it in childhood, usually just before puberty.
- OCD is also a very common childhood problem.
- Children with OCD have a better prognosis than adults, and the vast majority respond extremely well to treatment.
- OCD tends to run in families, but it is not a straightforward inheritance pattern. Both genes and life experiences may have a role in precipitating OCD symptoms.
- OCD is not a new condition, and historical figures throughout the ages have been described with what seems to be OCD.
- OCD can often appear similar to religious rituals. Members of a faith can generally distinguish when an individual is taking the religion 'too far'. Strict religious orders of any faith may attract people with OCD, but there is no evidence that religion causes OCD.
- It may be useful for therapists to work collaboratively with a prominent member of the person with OCD's religious group if he or she would like this to occur.

Reference

1. Karno M, Golding JM, Sorenson SB, Burnam MA (1988). The epidemiology of obsessive-compulsive disorder in five US communities, *Archives of General Psychiatry*, 45, 1095–9.

Chapter

3

Types and Presentation of OCD

OCD can present in many forms, but the most common symptoms of OCD feature one or more of a number of 'themes'. These themes will be described in detail and with the addition of case history examples. The main themes are:

- Contamination fears
- Fear of harm to others due to failure to act appropriately
- Fear of harm to self or others due to your own actions (or thoughts)
- Perfectionism
- Worry about losing something
- Symmetry
- Slowness
- Ruminations

The idea of 'magical thinking', whereby a person fears that by thinking a thought they make it more likely to occur, will also be described. Thought–action fusion, whereby a thought is believed to be morally equivalent to an action, will also be examined.

The final part of this chapter will examine other conditions which can occur alongside OCD, including physical complications arising from self-neglect such as infection. Other psychological problems and their relationship with OCD will also be explored and will include examination of depression, anxiety disorders, the obsessive compulsive spectrum disorders, autistic spectrum disorders, and schizophrenia.

Types of OCD

There are several themes which encompass all types of obsessive thoughts and compulsive rituals. The content of these thoughts may change over time in a person. The common themes of OCD also change depending on current news items and what is happening in the person's environment. For example, fear of contamination may frequently feature fear of HIV, whereas this would not have been the case prior to the 1980s. Similarly, someone who was previously concerned about general dirt and germs for fear of becoming ill may change this to specific fears relating to their offspring once they have children.

Contamination Fears

Contamination fears are one of the most common forms of OCD. In these cases, the person worries that either they will fall ill or they will cause others to fall ill, or they may feel 'unclean' and not 'right' if they believe they have been contaminated by dirt or germs. Some people fear specific infections such as HIV or bacteria that may cause vomiting, diarrhoea, or tuberculosis; for some people, the fear is a worry about general dirt and germs.

Case Study 3.1

Joyce is a 36-year-old mother of twins aged six years. Following a difficult pregnancy, the twins were born prematurely and had to be nursed in a special care baby unit. Understandably, this was a very difficult time for Joyce and her family as there was a risk the twins would not survive. Both twins did recover, and now they are normal energetic and healthy children. However, Joyce has an extreme concern that she might cause them to become ill unless she keeps everything in their home scrupulously clean. Consequently, she washes her hands up to 100 times a day, cleans the wood floors in her house with a diluted bleach mixture daily, and has a prolonged and exaggerated showering regime which takes up to an hour. She has been unable to cook for the children since they were babies because she is so fearful she might infect them. Fortunately, her mother lives locally and prepares the children's evening meal when they return from school and also their lunch when they are not at school. Joyce allows the children to pour their own cereal and milk in the mornings as long as she has disinfected the cupboard and refrigerator the day before. Joyce recognises these worries are excessive and unfounded, but she still feels extremely anxious.

The story of Joyce's OCD development shows how it arose following a very difficult time when there was a real risk to her children's lives, but now her fear persists and is mainly focussed on dirt and germs which she worries that she may spread to the children. She is able to trust her mother and others, including her husband and the teachers at school, not to infect the children, and she realises that her fears are both irrational and exaggerated.

Case Study 3.2

Mick is a 25-year-old man with a ten-year history of OCD featuring fear and avoidance of dirt and germs. At school, he was bullied for wearing glasses and being short for his age. He developed what he called 'self-preservation' strategies which were to always ensure he was extremely clean. Over the years, this developed into an extreme fear of his own urine and faeces and avoidance of any situation in which he might come into contact with other people's waste products, such as public toilets. Mick takes up to an hour to pass urine as he needs to ensure that no drop of urine has landed on himself or his surroundings. Moving his bowels takes up to two hours as he feels the need to ensure that his bowels are completely empty and that he is perfectly clean. Due to his problems, Mick restricts his food and fluid intake to reduce the number of times he needs to visit the toilet. Unlike many people with fear of urine and faeces, Mick denies he is anxious about becoming ill or spreading infection, but he explains his feelings of disgust about his bodily functions and how he feels 'morally superior' when he has completed his decontamination compulsive rituals to his satisfaction.

The story of Mick shows that very similar obsessions with urine and faeces can actually be related to very different thought processes. In Mick's case, his fear is very akin to that of people with perfectionistic OCD in that he fears being 'imperfect' or unclean.

Case Study 3.3

Marie is a 45-year-old woman with a long history of OCD dating back to her early twenties. The form this has taken has varied over the years. Initially, she had a fear of general dirt and germs, but during the past five years this has altered to a fear of contracting the HIV virus. In the past, Marie controlled her anxiety by drinking alcohol excessively to the point that she was consuming cheap wine or any other alcohol she could afford every day. While in a drunken state, she would sleep with men she had just met in exchange for them cleaning her bathroom and toilet. Five years ago, she had a health scare when she vomited blood and was told that she would die within five years unless she stopped drinking alcohol. She was sent for alcohol detoxification followed by rehabilitation, and she has been teetotal since that time. Once sober, she had an HIV test, which was found to be clear. However, Marie's OCD then focussed on concerns about contracting HIV. Avoiding public toilets and places where there might have been drug users (for fear of used syringes and needles), Marie began to limit the areas in London which she would visit. Her fear has now spread so that anything red, which she associates with blood, causes extreme anxiety. The local genito-urinary medicine clinic has asked her not to attend as she has been requesting weekly HIV tests.

The story of Marie shows how the content of OCD can change over time. She still has contamination fears, but these are now specific to HIV. Marie does not perform excessive decontamination compulsive rituals, but instead she tends to avoid areas that she fears may be frequented by drug users. She also avoids places where there may be openly gay people. In addition, she seeks medical reassurance by asking for repeated blood tests to check if she has HIV.

Fear of Harm to Self or Others Due to Acts of Omission

Fear of causing harm to self or others by failing to perform safety checks, or by failure to act, is another common obsessive theme. Some people fear their house may be burgled, which leads them to repetitively check doors and windows. Others fear they might inadvertently leave an electrical or gas appliance switched on which could result in harm and which leads to repetitive checking of electrical and gas appliances or even light switches. Some people with OCD assume extreme responsibility for others and may repeatedly report minor issues to the authorities.

Case Study 3.4

Ayesha is a 30-year-old married woman who has an eight-year history of fear that her house might be burgled. She lives with her husband and five children in a four-bedroom detached house in an affluent suburb. Her concern is that a burglar might enter the house while the family is sleeping or relaxing and that this will result in an attack on her children, her husband, or herself. As a result of this fear, Ayesha repeatedly walks around the house checking and pulling on the doors and windows to ensure they are firmly closed. Repeatedly checking in this way has caused her to break door handles on several occasions due to the force she uses. She even walks around the house four or five times each night after a prolonged session of checking before going to bed. These night-time checks tend to wake the family, and consequently the entire family is exhausted. Interestingly, Ayesha does not feel the need to check the doors or windows repeatedly when the entire family goes out together – for example, on holiday – as it is only when a family member is in the house that she fears they will be physically harmed. When on holiday, her symptoms tend to improve for a few days, but then she becomes worried about the security of the new environment and she starts to check doors and windows there.

Another example of someone with a fear that harm may occur is Amy (Case Study 1.2), whose fear of causing a fire by failing to switch off electrical or gas appliances led to excessive checking and then avoidance of using such appliances and reassurance seeking from her mother. Some people have more widespread fears.

Case Study 3.5

Mohammed is a 55-year-old man who lives on his own in a small flat. His mother, who is in her eighties, lives on an adjacent street. Mohammed worries that some type of disaster might happen to someone in his vicinity if he does not remain vigilant. An example of Mohammed's fears is that sometimes when he hears the squeal of car brakes at night, he will immediately leave his house to see if there has been an accident. If he does not find evidence of an accident (which has usually been the case), he travels to adjacent streets and often remains outside in all types of weather for two or three hours. He is well known to the city council for repeatedly reporting overhanging trees, loose paving slabs, and kerbs which he considers too high and a risk. He is also well known to the fire brigade for reporting any perceived risk of fire, including piles of leaves in the street. This overly zealous behaviour has led him to come into conflict with the police, who consider him to be a time-waster, and he has been cautioned for wasting police time. Due to his concern that he will get into further trouble with the police if he continues to call them, Mohammed now reports all his findings to his mother and asks her repeatedly for reassurance that he is doing the correct thing by not reporting them to the police. Mohammed's telephone calls to his mother can last several hours at a time, and he calls any time of the day or night. If his mother does not answer the telephone, Mohammed goes to her house and knocks on the door until he gets a reply. Once at the house, he generally refuses to leave until she agrees to accompany him to check on his latest concern. This behaviour is having a marked effect on an elderly and frail lady. Mohammed realises that the demands he makes on his mother are unreasonable, but he feels unable to resist.

The story of Mohammed shows how people who have severe OCD can come into conflict with the police, local authorities, or the neighbourhood in general. Whereas the underlying desire to prevent harm to others will appear an honourable one, the effect it causes in terms of wasted police time, when taken to excess, is also very clear. It also demonstrates how difficult OCD can be for the family of the individual. Mohammed's mother's health and well-being are being severely compromised by Mohammed's behaviour. When local health services had been involved, Mohammed was told that he should not call his mother more than once a day for a maximum of 30 minutes and should only visit her house at pre-arranged visits. His mother was advised to call the police if such unannounced visits were to occur, and to consider raising an injunction against Mohammed. As a loving mother, she had resisted doing this as she did not want to cause Mohammed to get into more trouble.

Fear of Harm to Self or Others Due to Acts (or Thoughts) of Commission

Some people have intrusive thoughts, urges, or images of a terrible event happening or that they fear they may have committed or may perform. These obsessions are similar to the sudden thought many people occasionally get when standing on a train platform to throw themselves in front of the train. The individual does not want to do this, but they feel as if their body may do it anyway.

A very distressing variant is images of harm occurring to loved ones. In these cases, the thoughts or images are very clear but are totally abhorrent to the individual.

Case Study 3.6

Sabine is a 20-year-old woman who was studying law at Manchester University but has had to postpone her studies this year due to her overwhelming OCD. A year ago, soon after she started university, she began to have vivid and extremely distressing images of her close family members being involved in an accident, severely injured, or terminally ill. If she learns about an accident while watching television or listening to the radio, she immediately has a picture in her 'mind's eye' of the same thing happening to someone she loves. Stories of beheadings in the Middle East have led her to have intrusive images of her mother undergoing the same fate. Similarly, she recently saw a poster regarding cancer research and immediately had abhorrent intrusive images of her sister, thin and emaciated and dying painfully from cancer. Although she realises that these types of thoughts are untrue, Sabine worries that her having the thoughts makes it likely that these events may occur. To guard against these terrible images coming true, Sabine will repeatedly say 'no' out loud whilst trying to imagine the same family member looking well or happy. Whilst performing these compulsive rituals, she will stand totally still and often remain in this position for up to 30 minutes until she can achieve an image of the healthy person without any 'traumatic' images. As a result of these symptoms, Sabine avoids watching television, listening to the radio, or reading newspapers. Whilst at university, she avoided mixing with other students due to fear that they might mention something which would provoke her compulsive rituals. This resulted in her restricting attendance at lectures and tutorials, and when the module concerning criminal law was timetabled, Sabine was unable to attend any of these as this would provoke more images. It was agreed with the university that she should suspend her studies until her situation improves, and now Sabine has returned home to live with her family.

The story of Sabine demonstrates a fairly frequent finding in OCD which is known as 'magical thinking'. Although realising this is not true, Sabine fears that having the abhorrent images makes them more likely to happen. Although people will recognise that such thoughts do not make the reality more likely, there are in fact minor variants of this 'belief' found in most cultures. Many people are superstitious about naming certain good or bad events for fear that by speaking them out loud or even thinking them, they can alter the likelihood of their occurrence. For example, people often try to touch something made of wood whilst saying 'touch wood' after stating that something may happen. The reason for touching wood is to try to 'undo' the negative impact that thinking or stating aloud an outcome may have. The vast majority of people do not really believe that stating an outcome will affect the likelihood of its occurrence; nonetheless, many feel compelled to act in this way.

In Chapter 1, the story of Jim (Case Study 1.3) was told. Jim has unwanted thoughts and fears that he may be a paedophile, and he spends much of his waking time avoiding anywhere there may be children, as well as checking that he has not had any chance to touch children. In reality, Jim is extremely different from a person who is a paedophile and would be a risk to children. First, Jim finds the idea of sexually abusing children abhorrent, whereas people who do abuse children do not find their thoughts abhorrent, and indeed will often have excuses as to why their behaviour is 'appropriate'. Second, Jim goes to extreme lengths to avoid children, particularly anywhere he might be alone and in close proximity to children. Again, this is very different from the actions of a paedophile. Due to the intensity of his thoughts, Jim does worry that his health workers have made the wrong diagnosis and that unless he can make them understand, he may uncontrollably grab a child, even though this is something he would hate to do. Due to these thoughts, he has occasionally tried to kill himself. Jim's entire history is different from that of a real child abuser. Unfortunately, people who have these obsessions can often be misunderstood when they claim they are worried about abusing children. In reality, people like Jim are almost the opposite of anyone who is a danger to children, because they will go to extreme lengths to ensure they are not.

Jim's story also demonstrates a phenomenon known as 'thought–action fusion'. This refers to an individual believing that having a thought is morally equivalent to performing an act. Although the thoughts of sexually abusing a child are totally repugnant to Jim, he still feels morally responsible for the distressing and hideous thoughts which come into his mind. In some religious teachings, it is stated that the individual must have pure thoughts to be free of sin. In the case of OCD, the effort of trying not to have these thoughts means that a person will have more of the thoughts. To demonstrate this, try to think about anything at all, but *do not* think about a pink hippopotamus *under any circumstances!* Once given this instruction, most people will immediately have an image or thought of a pink hippopotamus, and the more they try not to think of it, the more pressing it becomes. A similar circumstance occurs if you ever have a tune that you cannot stop playing over and over in your head, even when you actively dislike the tune and try to suppress it. You may try to not think of the tune, but the more you try, the more insistent it seems. The story of Eilidh also demonstrates how trying *not* to have a thought actually tends to increase its frequency.

Case Study 3.7

Eilidh is a 35-year-old woman who has frequent blasphemous thoughts which come into her mind and are shocking and abhorrent to her. Worried that these thoughts will result in her suffering eternal damnation, Eilidh tries to undo these thoughts by praying. She often spends up to five hours a day involved in these 'undoing prayers'.

Eilidh clearly has OCD, and the more she tries not to have blasphemous thoughts, the more they persist. Her story also demonstrates thought–action fusion as she believes that she should be able to control her thoughts all the time and that the more she tries not to have blasphemous thoughts, the more they persist and this is further evidence that she is 'evil'.

Perfectionism

It is not within human nature for things to be perfect at all times. Anyone who aims at total perfection in all things at all times is doomed to fail. Most of us can figure out when things are 'good enough' and will let that suffice instead of total perfection. It may be fair enough to believe in the old adage, "If a thing is worth doing, it's worth doing well", but when someone tries all the time to be perfect, the end result is usually extreme tardiness and failure to achieve very much at all.

The story of Geoff (Case Study 1.4) illustrates a person with perfectionism, who due to this became crippled and unable to perform much at all. When referred to the clinic, he had not bathed for months and was unkempt and in a poor state of health and self-care because he could not tolerate being just 'good enough'. It is clear that Geoff was far from perfect in his current state. As noted, this 'black-and-white thinking' in OCD is reasonably common. Someone who tries to have a perfect house may at times find it too much to deal with and end up living in squalor.

Perfectionism often results in extreme slowness. The issue of obsessive slowness is discussed later in this chapter.

Loss of Objects

Fear of losing items or even fear of losing part of oneself is another frequent obsessive fear.

Case Study 3.8

Ian is a 35-year-old man who works as a kitchen porter. Although he has a long history of minor and occasional obsessive thoughts and compulsions, he had always been able to control these and get on with his life until five years ago when his grandmother died at the age of 87. Ian had always been very fond of his grandmother and found it difficult to come to terms with her death. Soon after her death, he began to worry about losing objects. Mostly this has taken the form of worrying that he may drop things from his pockets. Before leaving for work, he checks his trouser and jacket pockets to ensure they have no holes. Indeed, as a result of his checking behaviour, he has created holes in some of his clothing. When his trousers develop holes, he does not repair them as he believes the stitching may not be as robust as the original. Once he places items in his pockets, he counts how many items he has placed there and writes the number on his arm in ink. If this number wears off during the day, Ian will become extremely anxious. He also places three tissues folded in a set pattern on top of these objects to prevent them from falling out of his pockets. Although still able to work, Ian is concerned that this preoccupancy is interfering with his concentration at work.

The story of Ian demonstrates the fear of loss of objects. Although this fear apparently began in his thirties, it appears that Ian has a long-standing history of minor obsessive fears. The story of Geraldine is another example of fear of losing things.

Case Study 3.9

Geraldine is a 45-year-old woman who lives alone. She has a long history of OCD starting in her teens when she would worry about inadvertently losing personal information which might be used against her. This fear developed throughout the years until she would not leave the house with any pieces of paper in case they might provide information which would be detrimental to her or her future security. Unable to express what information this might be, she remained very fearful even though she realised that this fear was unrealistic. Due to these problems, she has been unable to work as frequently as in the past because she feels unable to leave her house. She has also been unable to form close personal relationships as she fears that allowing someone into her house might result in her losing some information. Due to her inability to throw items away, she lives in a house which is in a severely hoarded state, and she is in danger of causing an avalanche of papers whenever she moves around. As she is living in a housing association flat, Geraldine is at risk of facing eviction due to the state of her property and the fire and health hazard it presents to herself and other residents.

Geraldine's story demonstrates how an imagined and unrealistic fear of losing personal information has meant that she now lives in real and tangible danger of losing her home and also placing her life at risk. This story also raises the question of hoarding.

Hoarding can be a symptom of many physical and psychological problems and will be discussed fully later in this book. There is also a condition, recently categorised as hoarding disorder. Unlike the situation with Geraldine, people with uncomplicated hoarding disorder do not have any underlying OCD fears, although many may have somewhat perfectionist personalities.

Some people go further than both Ian and Geraldine in their fear of losing objects and are unable to throw out urine and/or faeces without checking that they are not losing anything else first. This problem clearly has health and environmental implications and needs to be tackled with utmost urgency.

Symmetry

Problems with wanting to arrange objects symmetrically are frequently seen in people with autistic spectrum disorder which includes Asperger's syndrome. These topics are discussed towards the end of this chapter. Frequently, such apparent desire for symmetry in these patients is not true OCD as the patient does not have any obsessive thoughts but just feels uncomfortable if things are not symmetrical.

Issues with symmetry can also arise in people with OCD. In these cases, a lack of symmetry is usually related to an obsessional thought.

Case Study 3.10

Brian is a 30-year-old man who works as a shop assistant in a major electrical store. He is good at his job and was recently promoted to supervisor. Since the promotion, he has started to worry that a disaster might happen and that he might forget to perform an important duty which may lead to his being dismissed. In order to prevent this disaster from happening, Brian feels the urge to arrange all items around him in pairs which are exactly parallel to each other. To enable this to happen, there must always be at least two of every item in the store. Recently, he was reported to his manager as a customer wanted to buy a toaster. The toaster was one of two remaining in the store. If the customer bought the toaster, this would mean that only one toaster would remain. Generally, Brian will hide the single object until another one is delivered to the store. In this case, he was unable to hide the toaster because a new member of the staff was 'shadowing' him for the day. Brian refused to sell the customer the toaster, claiming it to be faulty. The customer asked to buy the second one, which Brian also refused to sell. Suspicious that something was not right, the customer complained to the store manager.

In addition to demonstrating how someone can develop symmetry compulsions, Brian's story demonstrates the paradox of OCD. Brian is fearful of losing his job, but by acting on his compulsions aimed to reduce this likelihood, he actually increases the chances that he will be dismissed.

Slowness

In the past, obsessive slowness was suggested to consist of purely compulsions without any obsessive thoughts. In fact, people with OCD do have worrying obsessive thoughts, although these may have become forgotten with the passage of time. Most people with obsessive slowness have a desire to be perfect.

Case Study 3.11

Lucia is a 19-year-old woman who lives with her extended family in a three-bedroom house. The family consists of three siblings, her parents, and her elderly grandmother. The house has one bathroom with a toilet in the same space.

Three years ago when Lucia was working towards her school exams, her mother noticed that Lucia seemed to be taking increasingly longer to perform simple tasks. She was working excessively and was taking longer to eat meals and spending a prolonged time in the bathroom. Her family initially thought that the behaviour was due to the stress of her examinations and that she would return to normal after they were over. In fact, Lucia performed much worse than expected on the examinations, and since then she has become slower in every action.

Currently, Lucia is unable to do more than basic self-care. Every morning she spends up to three hours getting dressed and then a further three hours in the toilet. Because it would take too long to complete, Lucia has not showered in months. Eating her meals, which her mother prepares for her, takes two hours, and so on many days she only manages one meal a day. She has started to restrict her drinking of fluids as going to the toilet takes her so long. The family is in crisis as Lucia's prolonged occupation of the bathroom and toilet means it is difficult for them to get to work. Her brothers often go to the local gym to shower, and the family has started using the public toilet in the local park. If anyone knocks on the toilet door, Lucia takes even longer to come out. Lucia says that unless she performs everything perfectly, she thinks she will be despised by her family and friends. She therefore feels the need to repeat every action until she is convinced she has performed it perfectly. If interrupted, for example by a knock on the toilet door, she has to go back to the beginning of her sequence of actions to ensure they are performed perfectly.

Lucia's story shows the paradox of perfectionism: In trying to be perfect, she is far from perfect and is a burden to her family. Indeed, the risk of being despised and arguing with her family is increased by her attempts to be perfect. Lucia realises that in trying to live up to her perfectionistic attempts, she is alienating her loved ones but feels helpless to stop. This story also emphasises how people with OCD can endanger their health by not eating and drinking sufficiently to ensure health.

Ruminations

Any compulsion can be either an action or a thought. For example, someone with contamination fears may either perform compulsive washing rituals or mentally go through evidence to disprove to themselves that what they have done is really a risk. When the compulsive ritual is an internal mental ritual, then the whole phenomenon can be described as rumination. Because this term often leads to confusion, I personally prefer to describe the content of the obsession rather than describe the OCD as 'rumination'.

Case Study 3.12

Billy is a 40-year-old man who spends up to six hours a day in obsessive ruminations. For the past 20 years, he has felt the need to rehearse his actions throughout the day at work to ensure he has not acted inappropriately or caused offense.

During the day, he works well as a clerk and is good at his job. He tends to isolate himself from his workmates and does not mix with them socially even at lunchtime and during coffee breaks. He isolates himself because the more contact he has, the more likely he is to worry he may have been socially inappropriate. Billy lives alone in a rented flat and has been unable to maintain friendships since the onset of his worries. Once alone at home, he replays every social interaction he has had during the day and repeats it until he can reassure himself that he has not been inappropriate or caused offense. This behaviour generally takes six hours but can last longer if he thinks he may have done something 'wrong'. He describes himself as lonely and wishes he had a family but finds that due to the worry which follows any social interaction, he cannot mix with friends after work, and it has stopped him from seeking a partner.

Ruminations often cause confusion. The problem is that ruminations appear to be a person just thinking the same thing over and over. Ruminations can occur with depression when the individual is consumed by negative and worrying thoughts. Indeed, just as slowness was previously thought to be an example of pure compulsions without obsessions, ruminations have often been described as an example of obsessions without compulsions or 'pure obsessionality'. In OCD, however, ruminations consist of two parts: the anxiety-provoking, distressing obsessive thought followed by the anxiety-reducing compulsive thought. It can sometimes be difficult to distinguish these two types of thought as they can happen in quick succession so that even the person with the OCD thoughts can become confused about the nature of the thoughts. Careful analysis in OCD, however, will usually reveal that there are indeed these two components. Only rarely does there not seem to be clear compulsions, but in these cases there is some other activity aimed at suppressing the thoughts which acts as an anxiety-reducing activity.

Are There Any Physical Risks in OCD?

Many people with severe OCD do neglect themselves and do not lead a healthy lifestyle, which can lead to a number of health problems or even an early death.

One of the most frequent complications of contamination OCD is that the person washes to excess. This breaks down the skin's natural defences against infection. Again with the paradox of OCD, people who fear contamination place themselves at greater risk of having a serious bacterial infection as a direct consequence of 'decontamination' compulsive rituals.

Self-neglect is frequently seen in severe OCD. Key issues which may arise from self-neglect include a risk of very low vitamin levels. As many people with OCD have restricted diets and spend a large amount of time indoors, low vitamin D is often found. This can lead to serious bone problems. Other vitamin deficiencies include vitamin B deficiency, which most commonly results in tiredness, and vitamin C deficiency, which usually causes an increased risk of infections. Many OCD sufferers who self-neglect do not have an adequate intake of iron, which leads to anaemia and extreme tiredness. A lack of fruit and vegetables in the diet leads to constipation. People who are worried about 'contamination' from faeces may deliberately make themselves constipated. Complications of constipation can include development of diverticular disease in which the gut becomes misshapen and prone to infections and impaction, which can be a surgical emergency when constipation is extreme and the bowel becomes completely blocked. If constipation is accompanied by excessive straining or excessive cleaning of the area, prolapse of the bowel, whereby part of the bowel hangs below the body, has been reported as a complication of OCD.

Another frequent problem with severe OCD is that the individual restricts their fluid intake either deliberately or because they are so preoccupied by their OCD that they forget to drink. In its most severe form, this can lead to irreversible kidney damage.

Many people with OCD go through periods of feasting followed by fasting due to their OCD symptoms. This generally can lead to rapid weight loss and weight gain. In addition, many OCD sufferers have restricted physical activity. Such behaviour can predispose individuals to an increased risk of diabetes, heart disease, and stroke.

Do Any Other Psychological Problems Frequently Occur in People with OCD?

Depression

Most people with moderate or severe OCD also have accompanying depressive symptoms. This is unsurprising when you consider how restricting and debilitating OCD can be. Fortunately, most people with OCD who are treated will also find their depression improves in parallel with the OCD symptoms. However, this is not true for a smaller but significant number of people who require additional treatment for the underlying depression.

Other Obsessive Compulsive Spectrum Disorders

Conditions such as body dysmorphic disorder, hoarding disorder, Tourette's syndrome, skin picking, and hair-pulling disorder are often described as obsessive compulsive spectrum disorders. Each of these conditions frequently occurs alone but can also coexist with OCD. These conditions will be described in detail in Chapter 8. When an individual has more than one of these conditions, treatment generally needs to address both areas.

Other Anxiety Disorders

Many people with OCD also may have another anxiety disorder. Generalised anxiety is most frequently seen. Fortunately, this can usually be treated in parallel with OCD treatment. Examples of anxiety disorders frequently seen with OCD include phobic anxiety and social anxiety disorder along with more generalised anxiety problems or panic disorder.

Post-Traumatic Stress Disorder

We have already seen that many people develop OCD after traumatic life events. For some people, these events were so traumatic that they have symptoms including vivid nightmares and flashbacks of the original trauma. Sometimes the OCD can mask the post-traumatic stress disorder (PTSD) symptoms, which can then worsen during psychological treatment. If someone has severe PTSD, such as can arise following childhood sexual abuse or following a traumatic incident such as a rape or a situation in which the individual believes their life is in peril, it is helpful for them to undertake treatment for the PTSD before moving to psychological therapy for OCD.

Autistic Spectrum Disorder

In autistic spectrum disorder (ASD), which includes Asperger's Syndrome, the individual has difficulty in understanding and interpreting the feelings and motivation of other people. This makes the world a very confusing place. Many people with ASD are more interested in inanimate objects than people as they find other people apart from their closest loved ones bewildering. Many people with ASD have stereotyped behaviours which can appear similar to OCD rituals. In addition, some people with ASD have the need for a rigid routine or for objects to be in a specific place. These symptoms, although appearing similar to OCD, do not have the same rationale as OCD. The individual does not wish to alter these.

In addition, a high proportion of people with ASD also have some OCD symptoms. The individual will, in the case of OCD symptoms, recognise these as troublesome and may wish to alter them. In these cases, the OCD can be treated in the same way as with a person without ASD, provided the therapist gains the person's trust.

Alcohol and Drug Misuse

OCD causes distress and anxiety. Some people seek solace and relief from anxiety by using alcohol, sedative drugs, or even illicit drugs to try to cope with the anxiety. Unfortunately, these are not the 'quick fix' that they may appear to be. Inevitably, increasing amounts of alcohol or drugs are necessary to achieve the same effect, and the person starts to suffer from complications of excessive usage.

Some individuals, most frequently with contamination fears, who wish to restrict their toilet visits may consume large amounts of anti-diarrhoeal medicines. This is also very dangerous. Anti-diarrhoeal medicines which contain codeine can lead to increasing escalation of the dose to achieve the same effect. Ultimately, these drugs can cause liver and brain damage.

Eating Disorders

Certain types of eating disorder have been particularly linked to OCD. Some of these individuals may not have a 'true' eating disorder but may be dangerously thin due to self-neglect. People who are starving often develop symptoms very similar to OCD. Thus, it is not surprising that some of those with very low weight due to a condition such as anorexia nervosa may also develop OCD symptoms. In these situations, it is important that the individual first gains weight until they are within the normal range before embarking on any treatment for OCD. This is necessary for three reasons.

First, as weight is gained, the OCD symptoms may disappear spontaneously. Second, any psychological treatment for OCD is stressful, and people with a tendency for self-starvation will tend to lose weight when stressed, which may be life-threatening. Finally, the drugs which can be useful for OCD do not work for people of very low weight.

Bulimia and obesity may also accompany OCD. In the case of bulimia, separate treatment for this is generally advisable before embarking on psychological treatment due to the risk that the stress of therapy will provoke worsening of the binges. Drug therapy may be helpful for both the OCD and the bulimia. In the case of obesity, treatment for OCD may help reduce self-neglect and improve the diet and increase the individual's activity once the OCD is less restricting.

Schizophrenia

A significant minority (approximately 1 in 10 to 1 in 25) of people with schizophrenia may also have symptoms of OCD. The incidence of OCD seems particularly common in people with resistant schizophrenia who are treated with drugs such as clozapine. There is evidence that in genetically susceptible individuals, clozapine can induce OCD. The problem is that clozapine is usually prescribed for people who have failed to respond to other antipsychotic drugs. Treatment with serotonin reuptake inhibiting drugs can be useful to control the symptoms of OCD. In a person with stable schizophrenia, psychological treatment of OCD may also be tried.

Personality Disorders

A significant number of people with OCD may also have obsessive compulsive personality disorder. These people have a tendency to be hard-working, perfectionistic, and frequently intolerant of others who are perceived as not living up to their high standards. This seeking of extremely high standards, unlike in perfectionistic OCD, is not seen as problematic by the individual. It is often difficult to clarify the extent of the personality traits and the extent of the OCD. In general, treatment for OCD should improve the distressing OCD symptoms. Sometimes people think they do not wish to change certain beliefs and behaviours but find that when undergoing OCD treatment, the beliefs they held rigidly are not as useful as they once thought and they can change with therapy.

Other personality disorders can also coexist with OCD. These personality disorders are frequently found in people who have experienced a difficult childhood. Emotionally unstable personality types are people who have difficulty regulating and tolerating their emotions. They may harm themselves through taking deliberate overdoses, cutting, or other self-harming behaviours when the emotions are too severe for them to tolerate. It is generally useful for such individuals to receive some help to try to cope with their emotions before beginning psychological therapy for OCD, although drug treatment may help the symptoms.

Key Points

- OCD often presents in several forms and with various themes described in this chapter.

- Magical thinking, whereby an individual believes that thinking of an event may make it more likely to occur, is frequently found in OCD.

- Thought–action fusion is also a frequent occurrence in OCD. In this, the person believes that having a thought is the moral equivalent of performing the deed.

- Ruminations are obsessions followed by compulsions, but the compulsion is also a thought rather than an act. The compulsion may take the form of a 'putting it right' thought or image which cancels out the obsessive thought.

- There are many physical risks and complications in OCD. These generally are caused either by excessive cleaning which can render the individual prone to infections or due to self-neglect. Other physical complications of OCD can be extremely serious and can range from prolapsed bowel due to excessive straining to kidney damage due to water restriction and a higher risk of diabetes, heart attacks, and stroke due to erratic eating patterns and lack of physical activity.

- Many other psychological problems exist alongside OCD. Depression, anxiety disorders, and other obsessive spectrum disorders are the most frequent. Harmful dependence on alcohol and other drugs can develop in individuals with OCD. Other conditions include PTSD, autistic spectrum disorder, eating disorders, schizophrenia, and personality disorders. Personality disorders may complicate OCD. People who have difficulty tolerating strong emotions are likely to find psychological treatment of OCD extremely difficult. In such cases, it is usually advisable to treat the emotional issues first.

Drug Treatment

This chapter starts by examining how, in the 1970s, the discovery that clomipramine, a drug used to treat depression, can greatly improve the symptoms of OCD led to the development of the 'serotonin' theory of OCD. Although clomipramine works well with OCD symptoms, it does have a number of potential side effects. The development of newer drugs which act on the same parts of the brain but have fewer side effects – that is, selective serotonin reuptake inhibitors (SSRIs) – will then be discussed in the section Serotonin Reuptake Inhibiting Drugs. This section will examine the possible benefits of these drugs and also discuss potential side effects as well as whether they are addictive and whether they can alter a person's personality.

We will then explore the options for people who have OCD which does not respond to SSRIs or clomipramine. This section will examine two main approaches to this problem. The role of dopamine blocking agents in OCD will be described. This will include discussion of how these act on a different part of the brain compared to SSRIs and clomipramine. We will then explore how some people with OCD fail to respond to the normally prescribed dosages of SSRIs but may respond to higher dosages. This needs to be undertaken carefully and with the close supervision of an expert.

The final part of this chapter will examine new research in the area which may be helpful for the future, including the possible role of drugs acting on the glutamatergic system of the brain.

Medication can improve the symptoms of OCD in six out of ten people. The first drugs that are likely to be given to someone with OCD are those which act on the serotonin system (Box 4.1). These drugs include clomipramine, which is an older drug, and the newer SSRIs.

History of Drug Treatment of OCD

Until recently, OCD was thought to be an untreatable condition. Many people with the most severe symptoms were in institutions. There was no description of OCD in the medical literature until the 1930s. People with OCD were offered

Box 4.1 What Are the Advantages and Disadvantages of Medication and Exposure and Response Prevention?

Medication is easily prescribed by one's general practitioner (GP). However, it can take two or three months before the real benefit is seen. There is little evidence regarding how long medication needs to be taken. The research evidence suggests that in many cases, it must be taken for a long time to prevent relapse. Indeed, some people may need to take medicine for the rest of their lives. In most cases, if a person has been well on medication for a year, it may be worthwhile to attempt to reduce or even stop the medication. This should be done gradually and with the guidance of a GP or psychiatrist. If symptoms recur, a person may need to restart at the higher dose again. Sometimes people can mistake the recurrence of symptoms as being due to 'withdrawal effects' of the medication. If medication is reduced slowly, there should be few, if any, withdrawal effects. The potential side effects of medication are described in this chapter.

Psychological treatment involving exposure is difficult. It involves commitment and requires the individual to face the objects, situations, and thoughts which they find anxiety-provoking or extremely unpleasant. For some people, this is just too difficult. Others find that they would prefer to take medication. Some people who find it difficult to face the fear may be helped by first completing a few sessions of cognitive therapy (see Chapter 5). Once people have learned the techniques of exposure and response prevention (ERP), then if they relapse in the future, which frequently occurs when going through a difficult time, they should be able to reintroduce some ERP for themselves before the symptoms become severe.

Some people will need a combination of medication and ERP treatment. These are usually people with more difficult-to-treat OCD who have not responded to either treatment alone. However, some specialists believe that it may be better to use a combination of medication and ERP from the outset of treatment with all people with OCD. This is controversial but is being studied.

sedative drugs to reduce their distress and anxiety. Electric shock treatment (also known as electroconvulsive therapy or ECT) was also tried for OCD, and although this is often extremely effective for some types of depression, it had no effect on obsessions or compulsions. More extreme treatments, such as a form of brain surgery called prefrontal lobotomy, reduced the symptoms of OCD but at the cost of a possible profound change in the individual's personality.

Clomipramine

A breakthrough in the treatment of OCD occurred in the 1960s and 1970s when modern-day exposure treatments started to be designed and applied to people with OCD with great success. At approximately the same time, it was discovered that the antidepressant drug clomipramine had a specific anti-OCD effect. This effect has been shown to be independent of and unrelated to its antidepressant effect. This finding led to a number of studies which showed that other antidepressants available at the time did not have such a beneficial effect on OCD. Clomipramine belongs to a class of drugs known as tricyclic antidepressants (TCAs), which work on a number of chemicals in the brain. TCAs have been demonstrated to work on the five major chemical systems in the brain which transmit information between brain cells. These chemicals are known as neurotransmitters. Clomipramine has a particularly powerful effect on the serotonin neurotransmitter system (also called the 5-HT system). It was discovered that clomipramine increased the levels of serotonin in specific areas of the brain. Clomipramine works by blocking the neurotransmitter serotonin from being rapidly taken back into the brain cells, resulting in an increase in serotonin. This increase in serotonin is believed to be the cause of the anti-OCD effect. The parts of the brain that are affected by low levels of serotonin in OCD are located in the front of the brain in an area known as the orbitofrontal area.

Although clomipramine is effective in reducing some of the symptoms of OCD, it is not without problems. Because the drug acts on a range of other neurotransmitter systems in the brain, clomipramine has a large number of potential side effects. The more common side effects of clomipramine include the following:

- Drowsiness
- Dry mouth
- Dizziness
- Headache
- Constipation
- Difficulty passing water
- Sexual problems
- Weight gain
- Blurred vision

Much less commonly seen are more serious side effects, including the risk of seizures. However, not everyone will experience side effects with clomipramine. The risk of experiencing side effects can be reduced by introducing the drug at a low dose with gradual increases.

Recently, concern has been raised about certain drugs used to treat OCD which may have a specific effect of slowing down part of the heart cycle, which extremely rarely may lead to sudden death in susceptible individuals. Clomipramine is known to sometimes cause this slowing, which is known as prolongation of the QTc. This can be checked by performing an electrocardiograph (ECG) test. Most people will not have this effect, and the ECG will be normal. Again, a gradual increase in the dose prescribed and monitoring by a doctor will prevent any untoward effects.

Another major disadvantage of clomipramine is that it is extremely dangerous in overdose. An effective dose for OCD is often up to 225 mg clomipramine per day. Rarely should it be prescribed at a dose greater than 250 mg per day, although occasionally doses up to 300 mg are used. An accidental or deliberate act of self-poisoning with clomipramine is very dangerous and can be quickly fatal because the drug can have devastating effects on the heart and other organs.

Serotonin Reuptake Inhibiting Drugs

After clomipramine was determined to be effective in treating OCD due to its effect on the serotonin system, drugs which had a more specific effect on the serotonin system without affecting other systems in the brain were sought. This led to the development of the SSRIs, which are generally better tolerated and have fewer side effects compared to clomipramine. SSRIs act on OCD symptoms and also have beneficial effects on depression and other psychological problems, including some anxiety disorders and eating disorders. Fluvoxamine was the first SSRI shown to be effective in the treatment of OCD. Although it has fewer side effects than clomipramine, fluvoxamine may cause slightly more side effects than the other SSRIs.

Initially it was thought that clomipramine might be more effective than the SSRIs in the treatment of OCD, but this has not proved to be the case, and there is strong evidence that they are equally effective. As such, there are few situations that justify prescribing clomipramine for OCD because the SSRIs are as effective, with fewer side effects, and are much safer in overdose. However, some people still prefer clomipramine, which is more sedative and also may help sleep.

Possible side effects of SSRIs include the following:

- Feeling energised, agitated, restless, or, occasionally, drowsy
- Feeling nauseous
- Not wanting to eat
- Difficulty sleeping
- Diarrhoea
- Dizziness
- Dry mouth
- Sexual problems
- Headache
- Blurred vision

Again, not everyone experiences side effects with these drugs. Unfortunately, it is not possible to predict who will experience which side effects with any given drug. Starting at a low dose and increasing slowly (every one to four weeks) tends to reduce the risk of experiencing side effects. Although some of the possible side effects of SSRIs are similar to those that can be experienced with clomipramine, the frequencies of these are usually lower with SSRIs. For example, problems with sexual function have been reported in up to 80 per cent of people taking clomipramine but in less than 30 per cent of those on SSRIs. Another factor is that the common side effects of SSRIs, such as feeling nauseous and not wishing to eat, usually wear off one or two weeks after starting the medication and do not seem to recur when doses are increased (Table 4.1).

What Drugs Are Most Commonly Used to Help OCD?

Table 4.1 Commonly used drugs for the treatment of OCD

Drug name	Trade name	Usual dose to be effective in OCD	Notes
Clomipramine	Anafranil	225 mg at night	This is an older drug which tends to be sedative and have more side effects than newer drugs.
Fluvoxamine	Faverin	50 mg in evening initially and increased gradually to 300 mg	Although it has fewer side effects than clomipramine, it may have slightly more than the other SSRIs.
Fluoxetine	Prozac	20 mg in morning and increasing every 2–4 weeks up to 60 mg	
Paroxetine	Seroxat	10 mg in morning initially, increasing every 2–4 weeks to 50 mg	
Sertraline	Lustral	50 mg in morning increasing by 50 mg every 2–4 weeks to 200 mg	
Citalopram	Cipramil	10 mg in morning increasing every few weeks up to 40 mg	Most evidence is for dosages of 60 mg citalopram, but it is only licenced up to 40 mg due to concern about specific heart slowing. (See 'Are These Drugs Safe'.) This means that it is possible to take a higher dose but that this will need to be discussed and in agreement with one's doctor.
Escitalopram	Cipralex	5 mg in morning increasing every few weeks to 20 mg	Most evidence is for dosages of 30 mg escitalopram, but it is only licenced up to 20 mg. This means that it is possible to take a higher dose but that this will need to be discussed and in agreement with one's doctor. At higher dosages, there is some evidence that this may prevent relapse of OCD. At higher dosages, there is some evidence that this may prevent relapse of OCD.

Do These Drugs Really Work?

No one can say that there is a perfect drug or that all drugs will always work for everyone. However, clomipramine and SSRIs do work. Approximately two-thirds of people with OCD will respond to treatment with these drugs. Most people who respond to treatment with these drugs have a 25- to 35-per cent reduction in their symptoms, but some obtain greater improvement. The tablets take longer to work than many people expect. Although helpful results can occasionally be seen earlier, many beneficial effects are not seen until after two or three months of taking the highest dose of the medicine. Improvements can continue thereafter, with further improvement up to two years after starting the medicine.

If someone does not respond to one medication, it is worthwhile to try another. It is not clear why some people respond to one SSRI rather than another, but it is definitely the case. Thus, for example, if a person with OCD has not improved on 60 mg fluoxetine, it can still be beneficial to switch the person to sertraline or another SSRI.

Although some people may eventually be able to stop treatment with SSRIs or clomipramine, those with the most severe conditions may need to remain on them long term. It has been shown that one in three people who have responded to SSRIs will relapse within a few months of stopping the treatment.

Are Clomipramine and SSRIs Addictive?

These drugs are not addictive and should not be stopped suddenly. They have an effect on brain chemistry, and stopping them abruptly can lead to a number of side effects. To stop the medication, it needs to be tailed off gradually over weeks. As such, this should be done under the guidance of one's doctor.

Are These Drugs Safe?

There is concern that people taking certain drugs may have a specific slowing of the heart rate known as a prolongation of the QTc interval, which is demonstrated on ECG. In turn, the concern is that a miniscule number of individuals with this abnormality may have sudden death due to heart arrhythmia. The development of these abnormalities seems to increase with higher dosages of drugs.

Drugs that are most commonly associated with prolonged QTc interval are those used as antipsychotics (discussed later), clomipramine, as well as citalopram and escitalopram. Sertraline seems to have the lowest risk of causing an increase in the QTc interval. It is advisable for anyone on an antipsychotic drug, clomipramine, or a higher dose of SSRI to have an ECG test annually and also when the drugs are changed.

Otherwise, clomipramine and SSRIs are generally safe drugs when taken in accordance with the instructions from the doctor.

Will Clomipramine or SSRIs Alter My Personality?

The short answer to this question is 'no'. As already explained, in people with OCD, there appear to be low levels of serotonin in specific areas of the brain. This shortage seems to precipitate the OCD symptoms. Clomipramine and the SSRIs aim to address this and increase the serotonin levels. Often, the individual's basic personality is intact but the person is free of the problematic OCD symptoms.

What Should I Do about Treatment with Clomipramine or SSRIs If I Am Pregnant?

This should always be discussed with one's doctor. In general, medication is best avoided, particularly during the first three months of pregnancy. However, the risk of relapse of the mother's OCD has to be weighed against the small risk to the baby. This should be fully discussed with a doctor, who should explain in detail the risks and benefits. In later stages of pregnancy, there does seem to be an extremely small risk of problems such as breathing difficulties.

Regarding breastfeeding, it is generally thought that the benefits of breastfeeding to both the baby and the mother outweigh any potential risks of drug treatment for OCD. Paroxetine and sertraline are the most commonly recommended SSRIs because they are found in lower concentrations in breast milk, thus resulting in low infant exposure. In general, when a mother is lactating, fluoxetine and citalopram should be avoided or used with caution because more of these drugs are passed onto the baby. This is not an absolute rule, and if the mother has been taking fluoxetine or citalopram during pregnancy, it is usually possible to continue to do so during breastfeeding with guidance from specialist medical professionals.

What If These Drugs Don't Work?

The most common reason people do not obtain a beneficial effect from SSRIs or clomipramine is that they have not been taking a sufficiently high dose for a long enough period of time. These drugs must be taken for up to two or three months before a beneficial effect is experienced. In addition to taking the medication in a sufficiently high dose, it must be taken regularly. Some people take the medication on sporadic days when their symptoms are most troublesome. Unfortunately, this does not work. The beneficial effect is dependent on a sufficiently high dose that is taken regularly. Missing one dose as a rare event may have no negative effect, but the medicine should be taken almost every day.

Some people fail to benefit even after taking the recommended dose of medication for three months. In these cases, it is worthwhile to try another SSRI because some people respond better to one SSRI rather than another. If this does not work, two other drug treatment approaches can be attempted.

First, and most commonly, drugs known as dopamine blockers can be added to the SSRI or clomipramine regimen. A second approach, which most likely to be performed by a specialised OCD service, is to increase the dose of SSRI above the recommended limit. Due to its toxicity, clomipramine should not be increased above the recommended dose range. A number of other treatment approaches have been suggested, but there is insufficient evidence to recommend these.

Adding a Dopamine Blocker

Unlike SSRIs, which act at the front of the brain, dopamine blockers act at an area towards the back of the brain which is linked to an area known as the basal ganglia (Figure 4.1). It has long been recognised that certain abnormalities of the

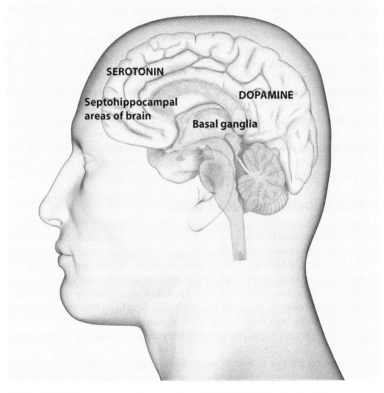

Figure 4.1 Diagram of areas of the brain targeted to treat OCD
Illustration © Dorling Kindersley; annotations by L. M. Drummond

basal ganglia and their connections can result in obsessions and compulsions. Examples include some movement disorders, such as chorea. In addition, the medicine used to treat Parkinson's disease (another disease of the basal ganglia) can also result in obsessions and compulsions. Dopamine is a neurotransmitter, but in the case of OCD, it appears that this is too active and needs to be reduced. The dopamine blockers bind to the nerve cells and dampen down the effect of dopamine. Dopamine blockers are also used to help treat conditions such as schizophrenia and other psychoses, and they are sometimes called 'antipsychotics'. The dose of drug used in people with OCD, however, is much lower than that used for schizophrenia. For example, it is not unusual for a patient with OCD to receive just 0.5 mg of risperidone with beneficial effect, whereas doses of up to 10 mg are more commonly used for schizophrenia.

Side effects with dopamine blockers are much less frequently seen than with the much higher doses used for schizophrenia. There is concern about the long-term side effects of movement disorders, but they are only rarely seen in people treated for many years with high-dose antipsychotic medication, and are much less likely to occur with the tiny doses used for OCD. Older dopamine blockers are known as conventional antipsychotics, and these tend to have more side effects. In addition, more acute movement disorders are sometimes seen with use of these dopamine blockers, but generally only at higher doses. Most of the dopamine blockers can also cause prolongation of the QTc interval, as discussed previously in relation to clomipramine and SSRIs. For this reason, people taking these drugs should be monitored by ECG. Aripiprazole, a newer drug, does not cause any heart conduction changes. Newer atypical drugs which have been used in OCD are shown in Table 4.2. In general, large-scale clinical trials of these drugs have not been performed, but there is evidence that they can be helpful. There is more evidence for some of these dopamine blockers than for others with regard to their use in OCD. However, the studies have generally all been small. Overall, there is probably more positive evidence for risperidone than for the others.

Overall, approximately one-third of people who have not responded to an SSRI or clomipramine will experience improvement with the addition of a dopamine blocker [1]. A large study also found that the addition of psychological therapy for OCD which comprises a form of treatment known as cognitive behaviour therapy (CBT) was more effective than adding a dopamine blocker [2]. CBT for OCD is described in Chapter 5.

Higher than Licenced Dosages of SSRIs

We have already mentioned that to be effective, doses of SSRIs for OCD need to be higher than those needed for depression. This observation that the improvement with OCD is correlated with higher dosage has led some people to prescribe above licence dosages of drugs. Of course, the upper limits of licenced drugs are sometimes overly cautious. It was previously noted that the licenced upper recommended doses of the drugs citalopram and escitalopram have been

Table 4.2 Newer atypical drugs which have been used in OCD

Drug name	Trade name	Usual dose for OCD	Common side effects	Notes
Risperidone	Risperdal	0.5 mg up to 1–2 mg if helpful	Drowsiness; dizziness; can occasionally cause weight gain	This is the atypical drug with the greatest number of studies to demonstrate its effectiveness in OCD.
Aripiprazole	Abilify	2.5–5 mg	Can cause an increase in activity and even anxiety; drowsiness is less common; can cause loss of appetite	This does not have any effect on the heart.
Olanzepine	Zyprexa	2.5–5 mg	Drowsiness; dizziness; weight gain common	Weight gain is common with olanzapine; therefore, this is not advisable for those who are overweight.
Quetiapine	Seroquel	25 mg	Drowsiness; dizziness; difficulty sleeping; increased appetite and weight gain	Weight gain is generally less than that with olanzapine.

reduced in recent years. Similarly, the upper recommended licenced dose of fluoxetine is 60 mg in the United Kingdom but 80 mg in the United States and several European countries.

One of the drugs which has been studied in higher doses is sertraline. Whereas 200 mg is the usual recommended dose for OCD, a study that examined patients prescribed between 250 and 400 mg found that, in general, they had greater improvements compared to those on lower doses [3]. For this reason, if an individual has not responded to SSRIs or clomipramine and has had adequate trials of psychological therapy (see Chapter 5), then the person can try a dose of SSRI above the normally recommended doses. This strategy, however, should never be used for clomipramine, which can be extremely dangerous at high doses. The prescribing of above normal recommended doses is most likely to occur in a specialist OCD centre. The ECG should be checked before each dose increase to ensure there is no change to the heart. In addition, it is often useful to check the blood levels of these patients.

In our centre, we routinely check the blood levels of patients who are on high doses. The most commonly used drug is sertraline. Despite dosages of up to 400 mg of sertraline per day, our results routinely demonstrate blood levels within the recognised range, and they are frequently at the lower end of this range [4]. In other words, although one might expect people taking these very high doses of drug to have blood levels at the high end of the range or even higher, our finding is that this is not the case. For these blood levels to be either within the therapeutic range or below it despite taking above normally recommended doses of SSRIs means that either these people have a problem absorbing the drug or they must rapidly break down the drug in the body. In fact, it often appears that these people rapidly break down the drug. Sertraline and similar drugs are broken down in the liver. It appears that some people have a very active metabolism in their liver and so break the drug down into non-effective components more rapidly than do the majority of people. These people are often described as 'rapid metabolisers' of sertraline or other drugs. This rapid metabolism may be inherited because certain genes have been identified which seem to be associated with this finding. People who are rapid metabolisers can be big or small, old or young, slim or obese. The ability to rapidly break down sertraline and other SSRIs is entirely unrelated to body size.

The Glutamate System

In addition to SSRIs and clomipramine, other drugs have been used to try to improve outcomes for people with OCD. Trials have been performed in which an SSRI was combined with other antidepressants, and some have used a combination of an SSRI and clomipramine along with various combinations of other drugs. Very few studies indicate that any of these methods can be recommended.

One interesting new area of research is the glutamate system. Throughout the brain, messages are sent from one cell to another via neurotransmitters. We have already discussed how in OCD, the neurotransmitter serotonin appears to be in the circuits at the frontal areas of the brain, and there seems to be an excess of the neurotransmitter dopamine in the areas connecting to the basal ganglia towards the back of the brain. The neurotransmitters are secreted into the spaces between cells by one neurone and taken into the cell by the next cell, thus transmitting the messages through the brain. Also in the spaces between the neurones are cells known as glial cells. One of the functions of glial cells is to secrete glutamate, which modifies the effects of the neurotransmitters. In short, the role of the glial cells and glutamate is complex and varies in different areas of the brain. In general, there is not a total lack or an excess of glutamate, but this may vary in differing regions of the brain. Glutamate is a modulating agent rather than a neurotransmitter.

Table 4.3 Drugs which act on the glutamate system

Drug name	Comments
Topirimate	An anti-epileptic drug which has been shown to have possibly modest improvements in obsessions in OCD
N-acetylcysteine	A modified form of a normal nutrient; may be useful for people with compulsive hair pulling (trichotillomania)
Riluzole	The first drug acting on glutamate to be tested in resistant OCD; does not currently appear to be effective, but there is ongoing research in this area
Memantine	A drug first used for Alzheimer's disease; preliminary reports suggest it may be helpful in OCD
Ketamine	An anaesthetic agent and a drug of human abuse; no evidence of long-lasting benefit in OCD, but further trials are being conducted
Pregabalin	A drug which has been approved in the United Kingdom for treatment of generalised anxiety disorder; may also be a helpful additional drug in resistant OCD [5]
Lamotrogine	An anti-epileptic and also mood-stabilising drug; preliminary trials in OCD have shown variable results
Glycine	An amino acid (i.e., a nutritional supplement); it has a low level of toxicity and may be helpful for some people

A number of drugs act on the glutamate system, which may be potentially useful in people with OCD who have not responded to normal methods. Clozapine, a powerful drug used in schizophrenia when standard methods of treatment are ineffective, has an effect on the glutamate system. In Chapter 3, we discussed how certain patients who appear to be genetically predisposed to do so may develop OCD symptoms after starting on clozapine.

Certain drugs which act on the glutamate system have been suggested as being potentially useful for OCD. These have not been subjected to extensive research and thus are still in the experimental stage. Examples of drugs which have been tested to determine if they are useful in treatment-resistant OCD are shown in Table 4.3. Further studies are needed before drugs acting on the glutamate system can be generally recommended for people with difficult-to-treat OCD.

Key Points

- Clomipramine was the first effective psychopharmacological treatment discovered for OCD. Despite being effective, it can have a number of disabling side effects and is also extremely dangerous in overdose. Selective serotonin reuptake inhibitors (SSRIs) were developed later and have fewer side effects.

- The following SSRIs have been shown to be beneficial in OCD:

  · Fluvoxamine
  · Paroxetine
  · Fluoxetine
  · Sertraline
  · Citalopram
  · Escitalopram

- Doses required for successful treatment in OCD are often considerably higher than those used for depression and most other conditions.

- Approximately 60 per cent of people prescribed an SSRI or clomipramine will have significant improvement in their OCD symptoms.

- The beneficial effects of SSRIs and clomipramine can take up to three months of regular treatment at full dose to manifest. Continued gradual improvement can be seen up to two years after starting the drug.

- Whereas some people may be able to stop treatment with SSRIs or clomipramine, those with the most severe conditions may need to remain on them long term.

- If an individual does not respond to one SSRI or clomipramine , it is worthwhile switching to another because they often respond to the new one.

- If two trials of SSRIs or clomipramine fail to produce improvement, there are two further strategies that are generally employed: adding a dopamine blocker or increasing the dose of the SSRI beyond usually recommended levels.

- Dopamine blockers improve symptoms in approximately one-third of people who have not responded to SSRIs or clomipramine. Adding dopamine blockers to an SSRI or clomipramine is less effective than the addition of CBT for OCD.

- Other drugs have also been examined to determine if they can help people who do not respond to SSRIs or clomipramine. Drugs that act on the glutamate system in the brain are one avenue of research.

References

1. Bloch, et al. (2006). *Molecular Psychiatry*, 11(7), 622–32.
2. Simpson, H. B., et al. (2013). *JAMA Psychiatry*, 70(11), 1190–9.
3. Rabinowitz, I., et al. (2008). *International Clinical Psychopharmacology*, 32, 49–53.
4. Vaughan, et al. (2018). *European Neuropsychopharmacology* (in press).
5. Leslie, et al. (2017). *European Neuropsychopharmacology*, 27(6), 620–1.

Chapter

5

Exposure and Response Prevention for OCD

This chapter will introduce the concept of graded exposure and self-imposed response prevention (ERP). It will describe the vicious cycle of compulsions and reassurance-seeking behaviours and the way they are rewarded by a reduction in discomfort. However, although these behaviours reduce discomfort, it is reduced only slightly, and the effect is often short-lived. Overall, therefore, the compulsions and reassurance-seeking serve to prolong and worsen the obsessive compulsive symptoms.

Avoidance of discomfort-inducing situations is also frequently found in OCD. This avoidance can lead to further worsening of the condition and an abnormal lifestyle which might, at its most extreme, threaten general health.

The treatment using ERP will be explained in full. Case histories explaining the principles of ERP treatment will be given. We will also examine the success and likely outcomes of treatment with ERP.

The reasons why an ERP programme may not work in any specific case will be examined, and tips for moving forward in subsequent ERP programmes are presented.

Finally, the role of other therapies, including cognitive strategies as well as counselling, psychotherapy, and family therapy, will be mentioned.

In Chapter 1, we examined the key features of OCD – the anxiety-inducing obsessions and the discomfort-relieving compulsions. We also examined how most of us experience obsessions and compulsions from time to time. We all know people who set extremely high standards for themselves. These people often have the obsessive traits of high achievement, meticulousness, punctuality, and extreme neatness or cleanliness. Indeed, traits such as striving for perfection and meticulous hygiene can be seen to have a survival advantage. This advantage may help keep these traits in the gene pool. However, in OCD, these tendencies have become an end in themselves, with the sufferer feeling compelled to perform compulsions even to the detriment of everything else in their life. For example, whereas general hygiene in the kitchen can be viewed as an excellent quality, in the case of an OCD sufferer, this may have developed such importance that every waking hour is spent cleaning the kitchen. For example, a woman with OCD and contamination fears had financial difficulties due to her inability to perform any paid work and also her excessive spending on cleaning materials. Both she and her young son were undernourished because too much time was spent cleaning to the detriment of actually cooking any food.

We also discussed how obsessions are thoughts, images, or impulses that appear in the sufferer's mind and are distressing and anxiety-provoking. Everyone has worrying or anxiety-provoking thoughts from time to time, but with obsessions they are so pervasive or so worrying that the sufferer feels the need to try to not have a specific thought ever again. Of course, the effort of trying not to have a specific thought means that the thought occurs more frequently. For example, a religious person may have blasphemous thoughts. These are abhorrent to the person, so extreme effort is made to try to prevent them from recurring. However, trying to suppress them is part of a vicious circle of constantly monitoring these thoughts and consequently increasing them. Much of the sufferer's time and effort are devoted to resisting the obsessions. Later in the illness, less time might be spent resisting as the individual learns this is not successful.

Common obsessions include the following [1]:

- Fear of contamination (particularly dirt and germs) due to the worry that harm may occur to self or others.
- Fear of harm occurring to self or others due to an act of omission – for example, fear that the family may be attacked if the doors or windows are left open, leading to excessive checking of these.
- Fear of harm occurring to self or others due to an act of commission. For example, an individual worries that they may run 'amok' and harm someone in the presence of knives. This often causes some fear in professionals dealing with the individual. In OCD, this is not a true urge or desire; rather, the sufferer does not want to perform the act at all and is frightened by the thought.
- Blasphemous religious obsessions. These are repugnant to the individual.
- Fear of loss of objects or inadvertent disclosure of information. For example, an individual may be unable to throw away household rubbish due to a fear that secret information may get into the wrong hands to the detriment of the sufferer. This can result in a house becoming virtually uninhabitable and filled with empty packets and papers.
- Hoarding. Recently, it has been recognised that many people with hoarding disorder do not have OCD. However, there is still a group of individuals who hoard objects for a variety of reasons related to their obsessional fears. For example, a man wanted to keep up-to-date on all book reviews. He therefore bought four newspapers a day and would repeatedly read over these reviews. He was unable to cut out the reviews for fear he might have missed some of the information. His house and garage were completely full of newspapers, and he had consequently rented a flat, resulting in financial hardship. The new flat was rapidly becoming uninhabitable due to continued hoarding of newspapers.

- Perfectionism is a common theme for OCD sufferers. Because nobody is perfect, these individuals are bound to fail. This failure leads to anxiety. Instead, the opposite of perfection often occurs, as the sufferer cannot even start to perform the action for fear of failure. For example, a woman felt the need to have a perfectly tidy house. She managed to achieve a pristine environment for a brief time. However, as the exacting standards became impossible to maintain, she was found living in squalor in an extremely anxious state.

- Symmetry was discussed in Chapter 3. These features can often be found in people with the developmental disorders of autism spectrum disorder and Asperger's syndrome. Some people with OCD also have a desire to ensure everything is symmetrical.

- Slowness, which was also discussed in Chapter 3, is usually related to perfectionism.

Obsessions are usually recognised by the OCD sufferer as being a product of their own mind. Importantly, however, obsessions are anxiety-provoking and often abhorrent. Therefore, an OCD sufferer who has obsessive concerns that they may sexually abuse young children will *not* do so. A true paedophile enjoys the thoughts of abuse and finds them sexually rewarding rather than repugnant.

In general, people with OCD realise that although very anxiety-provoking, their obsessional thoughts are either irrational or 'over the top'. After many years of dealing with OCD, this insight into the irrationality of obsessive thoughts can be blurred. In addition, if someone has recently been exposed to a situation that provoked their obsessions, they will at that point believe their obsessive thoughts. However, during periods of calm reflection, many people will admit the irrationality of their obsessions.

In Chapter 1, we also discussed compulsions. These are thoughts, words, or deeds which are designed to reduce or prevent the harm of the obsessive thought. However, either they are not realistically connected to the obsessive concern or they are clearly excessive. For example, an individual may feel the need to repeat prayers in sets of three following a blasphemous thought; the person may perceive this as a 'good' number. Thus, stopping at a number not divisible by three would cause further anxiety.

Sometimes, however, the compulsions are not connected with the obsessions in any logical way but, rather, are examples of 'magical thinking'. Most people have performed irrational magical, superstitious acts in order to prevent bad things occurring. In OCD, however, these behaviours are more extreme. For example, one man had the thought that catastrophe might befall his close family members. This was extremely anxiety-provoking to him, and he developed a compulsion which involved him standing on his right leg and hopping up and down in multiples of 12 until he felt that he had 'undone' the bad thought.

In addition to compulsions, some OCD sufferers repeatedly seek reassurance from others as a way of abating anxiety. This works in an identical way to compulsions. For example, whenever she returned home, a young woman had a fear that she might have inadvertently pushed a child onto the road whilst she was out. She would therefore avoid going out alone, insisting that a family member accompany her. Whilst out and on returning, she would constantly seek reassurance that she had not performed these acts by asking the observer to account for every movement and every minute of her time.

Although compulsions reduce anxiety, they do so inefficiently. They tend to reduce anxiety only slightly, and their effect is short-lived. For example, a man who has a fear of contracting diarrhoea from dirt and germs may wash his hands in a stereotyped way after every time he touches a door handle used by others. This activity will reduce his anxiety a little, but it will not be long before he believes he may not have washed his hands sufficiently well and he feels the urge to repeat his hand-washing routine. The end result is that people with OCD spend most of their time being highly anxious and distressed.

Compulsions are anxiety-reducing and/or discomfort-relieving activities which reduce anxiety and discomfort, albeit inefficiently.

The Exposure Principle for Treating OCD

Psychological treatment for OCD is highly effective, and the outcomes obtained with this treatment will be discussed later in this chapter. The treatments with the highest rate of success, however, involve facing the objects and situations which cause the obsessions, discomfort, and fear and to do so without performing compulsions. This may sound extremely difficult, if not impossible, to some people. However, it is certainly not necessary or even desirable to face all these at once. In any treatment programme, the person with OCD needs to examine the objects, situations, and thoughts which are likely to provoke obsessive thoughts. These are likely to range from those that are less fear-provoking to the most frightening. It is useful to then score these situations on a scale. I tend to use a 0- to 8-point scale, where 0 represents no anxiety at all, 2 represents mild anxiety, 4 represents moderate anxiety, 6 represents severe anxiety, and 8 represents the highest anxiety possible and complete panic. It is then possible to construct these situations into a 'hierarchy' or ladder where easier tasks can be performed first. These tasks should be performed without resorting to also performing anxiety-reducing compulsions. It must be remembered that old habits die hard, and many people find themselves performing compulsive rituals after exposure. This is fine as long as further exposure at the same level then occurs. Once an exposure task has been performed, the person with OCD will normally experience heightened anxiety for approximately two hours. This is normal in the early stages, but eventually the anxiety will naturally abate as long as compulsions are not performed. The key 'golden messages' of exposure treatment are as follows:

- Anxiety is really horrible and unpleasant, but it will not harm you.
- Anxiety will eventually reduce if you stick to the exposure task.
- Continued practice of the exposure task will mean that it becomes easier.

It has been found that to be effective, exposure combined with resistance of performing anxiety-relieving compulsions should

- be continued until the anxiety reduces consistently by at least a half (initially this may take two hours);
- be practiced frequently – ideally three times a day; and
- be performed reliably: The person should not move onto more difficult items on their hierarchy until they have mastered the easier ones. (Sometimes people are impatient, and while just starting treatment they will suddenly perform a task at the top of the hierarchy. This results in panic, and the individual can become disheartened and disillusioned.)

The treatment just described [2] is known as exposure and self-imposed response (or ritual) prevention or ERP.

Case Study 5.1

Eleanor has a ten-year history of fear of contamination by dirt from dog faeces. Her obsessional thoughts are that she might catch a variety of diseases, which could then be passed on to others and which would result in her feeling responsible for this plague. This problem caused her to avoid any situations in which she had seen dogs in the past. Even if she saw a dog through her window, she would feel anxious and resort to cleaning rituals. Her anxiety-reducing rituals consisted of stripping off all her clothes which were then considered contaminated and washing them: She would bathe in a set pattern and would repeat this ritual washing in multiples of four, which she considered a 'good' number.

Eleanor was seen in clinic by a therapist. Having obtained a full history of her problems the therapist explained:

> When you are in contact with anything which makes you feel 'contaminated', you experience extreme anxiety. A high level of anxiety is uncomfortable and so you will try to escape or avoid that experience. Escaping from the situation is not possible if you already feel contaminated. In order to reduce your anxiety you have developed the anxiety-reducing compulsive rituals of washing in a set pattern in multiples of four. When you perform these compulsions, your anxiety reduces. Because high anxiety is uncomfortable, this reduction in anxiety is like a reward. You are therefore rewarding your compulsive behaviour. If we reward any behaviour then we increase the chance of it recurring in that situation again. For example, if a dog sits up and begs and is rewarded with a treat, then you increase the chance of it sitting up and begging again. In the case of obsessional rituals, however, although they reduce anxiety, there are two problems:-
>
> 1. They only reduce anxiety a small amount.
> 2. The anxiety reduction is short-lived and you then have to repeat the compulsion.

> In practice this means that you are constantly experiencing very high levels of tension and anxiety. I am going to ask you to stop performing any compulsions at all. Although this sounds difficult, I think you will soon find that your anxiety eventually reduces much further than when you are repetitively performing your compulsions. You may on occasion find yourself performing your compulsions before you realise it. That is fine as long as you stop once you realise and then 'recontaminate' yourself.

This example demonstrates that the keystone of treatment for OCD is exposure to the anxiety-producing obsessions or the objects and situations which produce these thoughts. Self-imposed response prevention is also used as a way of prolonging exposure and removing the compulsions. The important thing to remember is that the person with OCD needs to face the fear in a reliable, regular, and graded fashion. In addition, the person needs to stop performing compulsive activities whilst facing the fear. The model for how the compulsions serve to worsen Eleanor's anxiety and how facing her fear without compulsions will result in reduced anxiety is shown in Figure 5.1.

Sometimes people with OCD make the mistake of also trying to produce a list or hierarchy of compulsions. Generally, this will not work, and it is often easier for OCD sufferers to stop the behaviour completely or replace the compulsive behaviour with a new, more adaptive behaviour. In Eleanor's situation, she would wash her hands and arms to midway between the elbow and wrist under running water and using antibacterial handwash gel. The performance of this compulsive hand washing would take three to four minutes, and it was repeated in multiples of four. She therefore had to be taught a new way of hand washing which involved putting the plug in the sink, using soap, and washing her hands to her wrists only for 15–20 seconds. (Singing the tune 'Happy Birthday to You' is sometimes used to time the hand wash because it is 15–20 seconds in length.) These new hand-washing activities could be performed whenever Eleanor went to the toilet or before meals. Her exposure tasks, therefore, were scheduled immediately after meals so that she did not reassure herself that she would soon be washing her hands.

Another problematic area was Eleanor's showering. Like many people with OCD and contamination fears, Eleanor did not take baths because she did not like sitting in 'contaminated' water. Instead, she would wash in the shower and then rewash her entire body in multiples of four. At the commencement of therapy, it was agreed that Eleanor should not shower but was to daily stand in the shower without washing for five minutes. A form of bathing that involved washing her body just once was also implemented but with the proviso that she leave one part of her body unwashed at each bath. Thus, one day she was instructed not to wash her right arm, the next day not to wash her left leg, and so on. This was done so that Eleanor experienced the idea of not being, in her view, 'completely clean'.

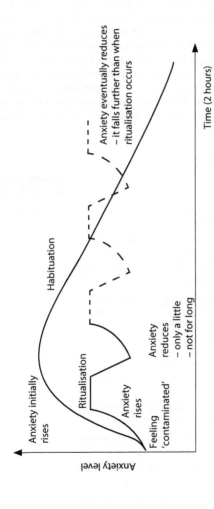

Figure 5.1 Eleanor's diagram

Reproduced from Drummond, L. (2014). *CBT for Adults*. London: Royal College of Psychiatrists

Eleanor set herself the overall goal of returning to her previous job as a fitness instructor. She had not worked for ten years due to her concern about dog faeces. In addition, she also wished to be able to go out with friends without fearing that she would have to return home if she saw something 'dirty'. She produced the hierarchy of situations to be tackled shown in Table 5.1.

In the hierarchy, it is noticeable that Eleanor was told that she would need to touch herself and also lick her fingers afterwards. This is because it is not effective if someone were to touch a feared item and then sit still not touching anything else until their next meal or next visit to the toilet to wash their hands. In such a situation, the anxiety is unlikely to reduce, and the person would not have fully engaged in the exposure. Similarly, if they performed compulsive washing rituals after the exposure, the anxiety will not improve in the long term. By touching herself and a variety of objects in her home, Eleanor was ensuring that

Table 5.1 Eleanor's hierarchy for ERP

Exposure item	Anxiety rating 0 = No anxiety; 8 = Panic
NB: All of the items are rated as if to be performed without compulsive hand washing and compulsive bathing/showering.	
Look at pictures of dogs and touch these pictures and then touch myself including my hair and lick my fingers.	1
Look at films of dogs and touch the screen and then touch myself including my hair and lick my fingers.	3
Go out of the house to the local shop and touch items such as the door handle to the shop. (Once I saw a woman with a dog excrement bag touch this handle.) No precautions and touch items in my house afterwards.	5
Touch my legs below the knee even though I have been walking outside as I fear they are closer to the ground and more likely to be contaminated. Without washing, touch myself including my hair and lick my fingers.	5
Go to the local park and touch the children's play equipment and then touch myself including my hair and lick my fingers.	6
Touch items handled by other people without washing and then touch including my hair and lick my fingers.	6
Touch the floor and then touch myself including my hair and lick my fingers.	8
Stroke a dog and then touch myself including my hair and lick my fingers.	8
Pick up dog faeces using a plastic bag and dispose of this in the appropriate disposal bin and then touch myself including my hair.	8

the effects of the exposure last longer and the anxiety reduces. Indeed, by licking her fingers, she was also ensuring that the 'risk' of her exposure could not be 'undone' by compulsive rituals. Of course, the term 'risk' is no real risk, and most people without OCD would have few or no problems completing most of these items. Some do seem extreme, however, and will be discussed later. This reduction in anxiety is also known as habituation. Habituation can refer to the reduction in anxiety following an exposure session which initially can take up to two hours. The term habituation is also used to describe how, when the same exposure task is repeated several times, the anxiety does not reach as high levels as before and does not last as long as it did initially. It is this habituation between sessions which can be used to record progress, and it is the reason why the exposure task should be repeated regularly (ideally three times a day).

Sometimes it is helpful to record the homework tasks in some type of diary. This can be as simple as a piece of paper or even a mobile telephone. The easier the diary is to complete, the more likely it is to be completed by an individual. For this reason, it is usually best to keep these as simple as possible. Such a diary only needs to include a list of the exposure tasks and the day and time these are performed. A rating of anxiety at the beginning and after two hours of exposure (without performing any compulsions, reassurance-seeking, or other safety behaviours) is also useful.

Why Some of These Exposure Tasks Appear Extreme and Not 'Normal'?

One of the surprises and criticisms people have when an exposure hierarchy is worked out with them is that it seems 'over the top' and that most people would not perform the acts that they are being asked to do. This is undoubtedly true, but the reason is quite simple. If a person has OCD and also fear and avoidance of certain objects and situations, once the therapy stops, there will be a tendency for the behaviour to return. If the person with OCD is still performing tasks in an obsessive compulsive manner, then this is a slippery slope which can rapidly return to OCD. I often describe the treatment as being like a pendulum, with one direction being increasing obsessional behaviour which I call 'OB' and the other direction 'slobbishness' or 'SLOB'. 'NORMAL' is in the middle of these two. If in ERP treatment we aim for somewhere in the 'SLOB' range, then when this treatment comes to an end and the person with OCD slips back slightly, they are still within a 'normal' range. Also, by performing tasks that are 'over the top', the person really challenges the obsessions and their veracity. Although most people with OCD realise that their obsessions are extreme and not based on reality, there can be a lingering doubt. Really smashing the obsessional thoughts by acting in a way so contrary to them and subsequently discovering that the feared consequence does not occur is a very powerful learning experience, and it provides a memory which can be useful if obsessions threaten to creep back into the person's thoughts.

Reassurance-Seeking

Some people with OCD use reassurance-seeking instead of or in addition to compulsive rituals. These people will repeatedly ask friends or loved ones for reassurance. Obviously not wishing to see their loved one distressed, most people will respond with reassurance. Reassurance, however, is similar to any other compulsive behaviour, and the more it is given, the more it is required.

Case Study 5.2

Katy is a 40-year-old woman who lives with her elderly mother. For the past 15 years, she has worried that she may have inadvertently caused offence to someone by something that she has said or done. During the past five years, this worry has increased so that she avoids going out except when accompanied by her mother. On her return, she repeatedly asks her mother for reassurance that she has not been rude or offended anyone. This can be repeated more than 50 times and can go on for several hours.

Katy's treatment involved a hierarchy of social situations which she faced up to. Her mother was asked to say, 'I'm afraid that I have been told by the clinic not to answer questions like that'. Over several weeks, Katy began to increase her journeys alone. At first, her mother had difficulty remembering not to give reassurance, but the more she managed to do so, the more she noticed that it curtailed Katy's demand for reassurance.

Katy's story shows how persistent and disabling OCD can be for both the person with OCD and their loved ones. Having a standard response available whenever her daughter asked for reassurance made it easier for Katy's mother to not offer reassurance. The fact that this response reminded them both that reassurance is not helpful in the long term, and that this had been discussed with them, may also be useful. Also, putting the onus on the clinic rather than on herself may have made it easier for Katy's mother to resist giving reassurance. Obviously, it is ultimately the responsibility of the person with OCD not to ask for reassurance. The person with OCD should agree in advance with their friend or relative how many times they can ask for reassurance before the other person gives the reassurance. This is because it is unfair for the other person to be badgered constantly, and the person with OCD does need to accept responsibility for their treatment. Needless to say, threatening and violent behaviour are totally unacceptable and should be dealt with in the appropriate way, including calling the police if necessary.

Reassurance can also be sought from other agencies, such as doctors' offices, or even by repeatedly searching the Internet. In the case of seeking medical reassurance, this is particularly a problem for people with health anxiety. It will be discussed in Chapter 8.

Other Examples of Treatment of OCD Using ERP

Contamination Fears

Case Study 5.3

Mike is a 30-year-old electrician who has always had minor obsessive compulsive difficulties. Five years ago, he was visiting the Metro Centre with his wife and went to the toilet. While in the toilet, he noticed some dried blood on the cubicle door. Following this incident, he became convinced he had contracted HIV from the blood. He visited his local genito-urinary clinic to have an HIV test. Unsurprisingly, his test was negative, but this did not reassure him, and so he started returning to the clinic on a weekly basis 'in case they'd missed something'. In addition, he became concerned about anything that he may have touched since he went to the Metro Centre or which he believed may have become 'contaminated' in another way.

These problems grew, and eventually he was forced to stop seeking reassurance from the genito-urinary clinic and his general practitioner (GP) after the clinic refused to see him again and his GP threatened to discharge him from his books unless he stopped making emergency appointments to see him regarding HIV. Although Mike was very anxious after this, the anxiety eventually lessened, but he continued to perform extensive 'decontamination' compulsions. These involved asking anyone who visited him who had been outside (and thus potentially in contact with somebody who may have been at the Metro Centre) to take off all their external clothes, which were placed in plastic bags. They were then asked to wash and bathe extensively. The clothes were sprayed 10–15 times with antibacterial spray before being washed in hot water several times. Clothes were often thrown away if he did not believe they were 'clean'. He had been unable to work for the past five years, and due to the stress of his compulsive rituals, Mike had started staying in bed for the past six months. Because getting out of bed resulted in so many urges to start his 'decontamination rituals', he was frequently incontinent of urine in the bed. In addition, he restricted his fluid consumption to avoid visiting the toilet. At the time of assessment, he was drinking only 500 ml of fluid a day. Bathing took him up to five hours; consequently, he bathed only once a month. His wife was tired and distraught and was considering divorce.

The first stage of treatment was to fully assess Mike and to determine his obsessional fear at the root of his problems. This was identified as 'a fear of catching HIV, primarily from the Metro Centre or from anyone who has been in contact with the Centre'. This fear resulted in extensive avoidance of leaving the house and extensive decontamination compulsive rituals concerning items which were brought into the house. In addition, there were widespread decontamination compulsions concerning the house and Mike's personal hygiene. Due to the extreme nature of these problems, Mike was avoiding basic personal care of washing and bathing. He was also restricting his fluid intake to reduce his use of the toilet.

The next stage of therapy was to ensure Mike understood OCD and the principles of treatment. It was described how he would be asked to face his fear and 'contaminate' himself without engaging in his 'decontamination' behaviours. The first issue that needed to be addressed, however, was his avoidance of drinking sufficient fluid. It was explained to Mike and his wife that such fluid restriction could lead to permanent damage of the kidneys. Although we would normally expect Mike to produce a hierarchy of fears, it was believed to be so important to address his fluid intake that any therapy would need to start by tackling this issue. Mike agreed he would drink 1–1.5 litres of fluid a day if he could use tissues to touch any item in the bathroom. Both the therapist and Mike's wife agreed to this, but he was told that he must also go to the toilet at least every three hours during the day to avoid any incontinence. Before the therapist saw him again, he was asked to produce a list of situations which would cause him to feel 'contaminated' and anxious and to give these an anxiety rating, with 0 representing no anxiety and 8 representing panic. It was explained that these anxiety ratings needed to rate how he would feel if he did not engage in any compulsive rituals or any avoidance to 'put right' the fear. Although he was initially allowed to use tissues when visiting the toilet, this was to ensure his health, and eventually he would be asked to forego the use of tissues.

Mike was very anxious about what he may be asked to do but did realise that his concern about the Metro Centre was 'completely over the top'.

At the therapist's next visit, Mike produced the following hierarchy of fears:

Exposure item (without washing/decontamination rituals)	Anxiety level predicted (0–8 scale)
Touch walls; door knobs; taps, etc. in house without hand washing after or decontaminating before	3–4
Touching clothes that have been outside	4
Using bathroom and toilet without 'decontaminating' first and by touching flushers and bathroom taps using bare hands	5
Walking to High Street and seeing other people; return home without changing clothes or bathing immediately	5–6
Travelling on public transport	8
Travelling to Metro Centre	8

At the next session, it was agreed that it was important to work on changing the compulsive behaviours and establish a reasonable self-care regimen. First, it was established that Mike had been drinking enough fluid during the previous week and was looking far less unwell than at the first meeting. Next, the therapist enquired about his bathing and the reason it took so long. As well as cleaning everywhere before going into the bath, Mike also had a set 'routine' of showering whereby he washed starting from the top of his body and worked down. If he believed an area had not been washed 'properly', he would repeat the routine. These repetitions often occurred eight or nine times so that each part of his body was red and raw. To break this pattern, the therapist instructed him to take a shower twice daily but that he was to stand under the shower for a maximum of 5 minutes and was not to use soap or try to 'wash' any area. He was also asked not to clean the shower before use. Mike agreed to try this and predicted his anxiety score for this activity would be 6 or 7. The therapist also showed him a new way to wash his hands (which could take 5–10 minutes) that involved plugging the basin of the sink and filling it a quarter full of water. 'Normal' hand washing taking 30 seconds or less was then demonstrated. This involved only the hands and not the forearms as Mike had previously been doing. Mike was then asked to try this with the therapist watching. He was asked to wash his hands only after going to the toilet and at no other times. It was agreed that at the next session, the therapist would visit Mike's house, and they would 'contaminate' themselves by touching items in the house which Mike believed were contaminated.

When the therapist visited the house, Mike was delighted to inform the therapist that he had bathed in the prescribed fashion all week, continued to maintain his fluid levels, and washed his hands as demonstrated. The therapist praised him and then demonstrated how Mike should expose himself to 'contamination'. This involved touching the 'contaminated' object with both hands; rubbing the hands together and then touching his hair, upper torso, lower torso, legs, lips, and mouth; and then licking his hands to ensure that he felt 'contaminated'. Mike was extremely anxious about this but was reminded of the habituation curve and agreed to give it a try. In fact, he did extremely well, and during the session he agreed to go further and touch the toilet flusher and taps without washing. He was praised and was asked to continue performing these exposure exercises three times a day for the next week.

Treatment continued in this way. Mike was asked to touch the toilet seat and contaminate himself in the prescribed manner. The principle of performing tasks which appear excessive was discussed previously. It is often useful to overlearn these tasks to prevent reversion to previous behaviours after therapy ends.

After nine sessions, Mike agreed to accompany the therapist to the Metro Centre. They travelled around the Metro Centre, touching as many items as possible. They went into the toilets and touched the taps and toilet flushers and the door. Then they went to the burger shop and ate a burger without washing their hands. Mike was anxious, but he settled as the day progressed. This exposure session lasted a total of four hours, including travel on public transport to get to the Metro Centre.

Is ERP Dangerous?

Some people worry that exposure exercises such as those described previously are 'risky' and that it is unethical to ask someone to risk contracting an illness by not washing. The risk of contracting HIV by such activity is almost zero, but there is a very small possibility of contracting another less serious infection. It is important to remember, however, that all of us perform risky behaviours every day when we drive a car or cross a road on foot. Patients with OCD can be restricted in all aspects of their lives for decades. If asked to weigh the tiny risk of catching a minor illness against suffering from OCD with its life-impacting consequences, most people will conclude that the risk of ERP is overshadowed by the life-destroying effects of OCD.

It must also be remembered that the body has protection to fight infection. The skin forms a thick barrier to infection. It is covered with normal helpful bacteria which help prevent harmful bacteria from spreading. Excessive washing, as seen in many people with OCD and decontamination compulsions, actually destroys some of these bacteria and can make skin infection more likely. The use of antibacterial gels and sprays (or, even worse, antiseptics and bleach) adds to this effect and greatly increases the risk of infection. Excessive washing also serves to thin the skin, and many people with hand-washing compulsive rituals have open cuts and sores on their hands and other parts of their bodies where they wash excessively. This results in a direct route for infection into the body and also greatly increases the risk of infection. In fact, studies have been performed at the University of Sydney whereby people were asked to touch things commonly perceived as 'dirty' by people with contamination OCD. When hands that touched these 'dirty' items were compared with hands that did not touch these items, there were no differences in the types and numbers of bacteria. This finding is part of the 'evidence' presented to people who undertake danger ideation reduction therapy (discussed later).

Indeed, the best hand-washing technique in most normal situations is to wash hands for the duration it takes to sing 'Happy Birthday to You' in one's head or, in other words, for 15–30 seconds.

Treatment of Checking Compulsions

Case Study 5.4

Jill is a 30-year-old woman with a 10-year history of minor obsessive fears. Five years ago, she moved away from her parental home into her own studio flat and started a new job as a legal secretary. Since moving into her flat, Jill has become very anxious that a disaster will occur, resulting in her losing all her belongings. She therefore feels the need to check her cooker and all electrical appliances to ensure they are switched off and repeatedly checks her doors and windows before leaving for work. Initially, these checks took only a few minutes, but the time required has gradually increased so that they currently take up to two hours. Recently, she has even become concerned about leaving the freezer on whilst she is out. Having had a minor flood in her flat and being forced to throw food away, she has emptied the freezer and now only uses the refrigerator as a store for milk and butter and switches this off when not in the house. Realising that this problem is getting out of control, Jill decide to seek help.

Jill's problems were still under control but were starting to impact her ability to work as well as her ability to feed herself because she needed to buy fresh food every day. Initially, she set up a hierarchy of her fears, which were as follows:

Exposure item	Anxiety rating (0–8 scale)
Not checking light switches when leaving the flat	2
Not checking television and computer are switched off when leaving the flat	3
Not checking the refrigerator	4
Leaving the refrigerator and freezer switched on whilst leaving flat	5
Not checking hair straighteners when leaving flat	6
Not checking windows when leaving flat	7
Not checking front door when leaving flat	8

It was decided that Jill would start therapy herself by not checking light switches, television, and the computer when leaving the flat. She easily performed these tasks but then became stuck. Feeling just too scared to move on to the other items on her hierarchy, Jill believed she could not move forward. It was agreed that she would take a day off work and meet with the therapist. On the day she was to do this, Jill was to get ready to go out but was not to check any of the items on her hierarchy. She would telephone the therapist on her mobile phone, who talked her through walking out of the flat without checking. Jill would then travel to the clinic with the risk that a disaster had happened to her possessions.

Although this was a difficult exercise, Jill managed to complete it. She was tearful and shaking whilst at the clinic, but this settled after two hours. During this time, she was encouraged to think of the 'worst-case scenario' whereby she returned home to find her flat burgled or burned to the ground. Following this session, Jill has been able to continue this regimen on a daily basis. Some days are more difficult than others and she has a stronger urge to check, but despite a few setbacks, she persists and finds that her overall anxiety is reduced to mild levels.

Perfectionism and Slowness

Case Study 5.5

Colin is a 45-year-old man who lives with his wife and two children. He previously worked as a clerk for a building firm but had to leave this job five years ago due to an inability to complete his work on time. Since being at home, he has become increasingly slower at performing a range of tasks so that now he can take up to six hours in the bathroom. This problem impacts the family, and he has recently started sleeping during the day and waking at night to avoid restricting family access to the bathroom due to his OCD. Colin believes that everything he does needs to be performed 100 per cent correctly or else he will be a failure. Being a failure means that his family and friends will abandon him. In discussion, he agrees that he is more 'fussy' that other people. Although he still likes the idea of being 'perfect', he realises that he is far from it in his current state and is thus willing to try to change and to be 'good enough'. The first phase of this treatment is to deliberately perform actions incorrectly. Colin believed he would like to start with this problem rather than tackle his bathing and toileting problems (even though this means he has to attend the clinic having had little sleep). Colin produced the following list of 'wrong' items and the anxiety they would cause:

Exposure item	Anxiety rating (0–8 scale)
Wearing odd socks all day	3
Wearing T-shirt inside out and back to front	4
Making a cup of tea and adding the milk first (Colin believes the milk should always be added afterwards, although he realises others disagree.)	4
Leaving one arm unwashed in the shower	3
Leaving one leg unwashed in the shower	4
Not combing hair	4
Shaving with electrical razor without looking in mirror	4
Eating dessert before main course	3

Because Colin may be tempted to perform each of these exposure items perfectly, he was instructed that as soon as he got up he was to throw a die three times until he obtained three different numbers. The three numbers represented the three items that he had to perform each day. He was to continue otherwise as normal. In addition, he was asked to only perform his programme 75 per cent correctly rather than strive to be the 'perfect patient'.

Colin managed to perform the 'imperfect' programme with approximately 70 per cent compliance. He performed all the items on the list several times over a few weeks. However, he was still spending many hours in the bathroom before being able to get out and was also spending up to two hours in the toilet every time he went to pass water. Colin stated that the reason he took so long was that he felt the need to perform tasks until they felt 'just right'. This involved, for example, sitting on the toilet seat and altering his position several times over many minutes until he felt he was completely balanced and symmetrical. Because the list of items such as these that Colin performed was so numerous, it was agreed to tackle this in one go. The therapist agreed to visit Colin's home for a morning and talk him through getting up and dressed in no more than two hours. Before this meeting, Colin had been asked to practice items such as sitting asymmetrically on the toilet seat.

When the therapist arrived at Colin's house, he was dressed in his pyjamas. The first task was to get him to eat his breakfast. Every day, Colin's breakfast consisted of cereal and milk with a cup of tea. He was encouraged to sit down and, without arranging his cutlery perfectly next to the cereal bowl, pour the approximate amount of cereal and milk he required without measuring these. Then he was to drink his tea rapidly. He was to perform these eating and drinking activities without a break to ensure he was doing them correctly. Once he had eaten, he needed to go to the toilet and shower. Obviously, the therapist did not accompany him but, rather, remained outside the bathroom and encouraged Colin to sit imperfectly on the toilet seat and to take a shower without checking that he washed every part of his body perfectly. It was decided that he should then get dressed before shaving. Colin would normally check that his clothes were perfectly ironed and would make sure that he put them on his body so that they were perfectly straight. He was encouraged to take a risk and put his clothes on in a more 'haphazard' manner before moving on to shaving and brushing his hair. Shaving was to take no more than four minutes and hair brushing 30 seconds. Colin found hair brushing very difficult as he tried to copy the technique of the therapist, who showed Colin how he brushed his hair.

The entire process took two hours. Colin said that he did not feel 'right' following this but was happy to continue. The therapist had made an audio recording of the entire session on Colin's mobile phone. Colin was asked to listen to the recording every day for the next week and to keep to the schedule.

When Colin returned to see the therapist a week later, he had not only achieved this goal but also was taking less than one hour and so had abandoned the tape. He was taking only five minutes to go to the toilet during the day and was feeling much happier.

Currently, Colin is still aware that he occasionally has urges to be 'perfect' but mostly manages to resist these. He is happier and is going out with his family without demanding that they perform actions perfectly as well. He is thinking about attending adult education classes to retrain as a gardener.

Colin's story again demonstrates the main principle of treating OCD by using ERP. In Colin's situation, his basic fear is the consequence of being less than perfect. Therapy was designed to encourage him to perform actions imperfectly and, by so doing, find out what happens when he is 'imperfect'. In reality, of course, all of us are imperfect, and in Colin's case, his constant seeking for perfection meant that he was able to do very little and was thus far from perfect as an employee (he had to stop working), as a father (he rarely saw his children), and as a husband (he rarely saw his wife and was unable to be a 'partner' in the relationship). Once he abandoned striving for perfection, he was much more successful in all areas of his life.

Obsessions with Covert Compulsions (Ruminations)

People often become confused about so-called obsessive ruminations. This is because they are used to the idea that anxiety-provoking obsessive *thoughts* are followed by anxiety-reducing compulsive *behaviours*. However, compulsions can be behaviours, thoughts, or images. As such, any ERP therapy must identify the anxiety-provoking thoughts whilst stopping the anxiety-reducing compulsive thoughts.

Case Study 5.6

Ethan, a 42-year-old unmarried ex-schoolteacher, has a 15-year history of distressing obsessions which occupied 10–12 hours a day and led to his early retirement from work. Whenever he saw anyone, he would have the thought, 'I would like to have sex with him/her'. This thought was repugnant to him because he was a devout 'born-again' Christian who did not condone extramarital sex and because homosexuality, paedophilia, and incest, which his thoughts implied, were abhorrent to him.

To reduce his anxiety, he had developed the habit of repeating the Lord's Prayer and then saying 'Jesus, forgive me' seven times. If he was interrupted by any sound or movement in his environment, he would have to repeat this process until it was performed perfectly. This problem led him to seek the life of a recluse, and he had even stopped attending church. He had contemplated suicide to rid himself of the problem, but he believed this was an even greater sin.

Initially, treatment took the form of graduated prolonged exposure to situations he avoided. However, he made only limited progress because he could not stop himself from automatically starting his 'praying ritual' which helped to maintain his anxiety. It was decided that he needed to experience prolonged exposure to his anxiety-provoking thoughts without ritualising. This was achieved by having him record these thoughts (e.g., 'I want to have sex with her' and 'I want to have sex with him') on his smartphone. Ethan was then asked to play these thoughts to himself via the phone's earpiece for at least one hour three or four times a day while in the company of other people (e.g., while riding the bus).

Initially, Ethan found this so aversive that he had difficulty complying. There-fore, the therapist advised him to start with the volume turned down low and to increase the volume as he became more confident. This procedure worked extremely well, and within two weeks, Ethan reported that he had little anxiety and was able to go out at other times and not just when performing his pro-grammes. Despite having the thoughts, he no longer carried out the ritual. After two months, he was able to return to work as a 'supply' teacher. At six-month post-treatment follow-up, he reported that he had a girlfriend, he was planning to marry, and he laughed at the thoughts which he now considered to be 'stupid'.

Two issues appear to be of particular importance in this treatment. First, it appears to be most effective if the recording is made by the person with OCD rather than by another person. Second, it appears to be more effective if it is played through an earpiece. The effect of these two is that it seems virtually impossible for the person with OCD to perform compulsive thought rituals whilst their own voice is repeating the obsessive thought. The fact that it is their own voice and is heard in their head means it is difficult to concentrate on much else initially.

Treatment of OCD with Hoarding Problems

Hoarding disorder will be fully discussed in Chapter 8. The symptom of hoarding, however, can occur in people with OCD. Joan's story illustrates how hoarding can be part of OCD and how it can be tackled.

Case Study 5.7

Joan is a 42-year-old woman who lives with her husband and two teenaged chil-dren. She has suffered from a series of obsessive worries all her life, but these had not been overly problematic until the birth of her youngest child 15 years ago. This had been a difficult delivery, and Joan had suffered massive bleeding during labour. There was concern about the baby, and he was taken to the paediatric inten-sive care unit overnight. Although there was no long-lasting effect on his health, Joan understandably found this to be a very difficult experience. Following the birth, she developed postnatal depression. This depression was eventually noted and treated with antidepressants nine months after the birth, but Joan was left with residual obsessive fears. Joan fears that she may inadvertently disclose infor-mation which will lead to her losing her children. She is not worried about verbally giving away information but, rather, that she may write something down which is incriminating and, as a written word, would be more difficult to explain away.

Initially, this problem meant that Joan felt the need to meticulously check all pieces of paper in the house for fear they may contain some detrimental information. All labels, receipts, letters, and papers which came into the house were repeatedly checked. During the past 8 years, this problem has become increasingly worse, and Joan is now unable to throw out any written material, including empty food packets. The family lives in a large detached four-bedroomed house, but it is quickly becoming uninhabitable due to Joan's hoarding. Initially, the double garage was filled from floor to ceiling, but now the spare bedroom is becoming full and Joan wants her sons to share a bedroom so that she can continue to hoard her items. During the past 3 years, in addition to paper items, Joan has also been collecting pieces of paper and detritus left on the pavement in case these also contain damaging revelations about her. Joan realises that these thoughts are ridiculous and untrue, and she also realises the stress she is causing the family, but she still has an overwhelming fear when faced with pieces of paper.

When Joan came to the clinic and discussed her problem, it was agreed that the first issue to be tackled would be working on preventing more items from being brought into the house. With anybody who hoards, it must first be established that no more items will be brought into the house while the clearing of items is taking place. Otherwise, the exercise of clearing the house is pointless because the hoard will rapidly reaccumulate. Obviously, in a situation such as Joan's, some items will continue to come into the house in the form of letters and food packaging. It was thus decided that therapy would start with an exposure programme involving Joan's fear of revealing information. It was very difficult for Joan to create a hierarchy of her fears because all related to her fear of revealing detrimental information. Throwing away a food packet was as anxiety-provoking as throwing away a piece of paper with her writing on it because she believed both may contain damaging information. Eventually, it was agreed that the therapist would write out times on several pieces of paper, 'I declare that I am a bad mother and that my children should be taken away from me'. These pieces of paper were then signed by the therapist. This exercise was designed to be anxiety-provoking for Joan but also demonstrated that the therapist was prepared to take the same or greater risk herself. Joan and the therapist then walked into the main High Street of town and deposited these pieces of paper in litter bins, on a table in a fast-food restaurant, and on a table in a local library. Joan found this very anxiety-provoking but agreed that she would not return to the High Street to collect these papers later. She also agreed to go out every day and to throw away blank pieces of paper in the way the therapist and she had done during the session.

The next week, Joan was feeling very pleased and had already been able to throw away printed paper. She was praised for doing so. It was agreed that in light of this, therapy should move on to throwing away some of the hoarded items. Initially, Joan wanted to check all the papers she threw away. The therapist reminded her that this checking was likely to lead to more checking and more anxiety. Eventually, she agreed to start throwing away items in the garage which had been there for more than two years. During the first session, the therapist and Joan managed to discard six large rubbish sacks full of paper. Joan agreed to let the therapist take these to the local tip so that she could not check them later. She also agreed to put out at least two sacks per day for her husband to discard on his way to work.

Over the next few weeks, Joan cleared most of her house. Dealing with newer post was difficult initially, but she was reminded of the principle that she should read any post, act on it immediately if necessary, and then discard it.

Does ERP Really Work?

Studies throughout the years [3] have repeatedly shown that approximately 75 per cent of people with OCD who are offered ERP will improve. The rate of improvement is generally measured using a scale known as the Yale–Brown Obsessive–Compulsive Scale (Y-BOCS). To be identified as a 'responder' to either drugs or ERP (see Box 4.1), an improvement of more than 35 per cent on the Y-BOCS should be found from the start of treatment to the end of treatment. In reality, this is probably an underestimate because the Y-BOCS is not very sensitive to anything other than large improvements in symptoms. An improvement of 35 per cent on the Y-BOCS is often found to be accompanied by an improvement in life functioning of 50 per cent or more.

It has proven impossible to predict precisely who responds the most to treatment with ERP. Certainly children appear to respond better than adults. Obviously, if a person has had a mild problem for a short time, they may also be expected to respond well to treatment. However, this is not an absolute rule. Many people who have had profound OCD problems for many decades can still respond to ERP. This may be because they are more motivated to carry out the treatment to overcome the OCD which has blighted their lives. A study involving some of the most profoundly ill people treated in our inpatient ward and severely ill people treated in the community examined outcomes and found few clear predictors of success at the beginning of treatment [4].

The main factor which determines how much improvement a person can gain from ERP seems to be how well they can adhere to the treatment programmes and face their fears without the anxiety-relieving compulsions.

What Are the Reasons Why ERP May Not Work?

There are several very obvious reasons why ERP may not work. First, the person has to be committed to change. If they do not wish to stop the OCD then, obviously, they will not be motivated to apply the treatment. It is often extremely difficult for the family and friends of someone with OCD to understand why the person with OCD would not want to overcome this potentially devastating condition. Humans generally dislike change and tend to feel secure with what they know. Asking someone to give up the OCD symptoms, which are so familiar to them, can feel threatening and scary. Sometimes the treatment can seem worse than the OCD. Indeed, OCD seems to give some individuals comfort and security; losing the label of OCD would mean that they have to face the problems of the world, such as working for a living, moving out of the parental home, or forming new relationships. In this case, OCD gives them a reason to not engage with these challenges. When a person with OCD does not wish to change, then ERP will not work. Very often, friends and relatives of the person with OCD believe that the therapists have failed their loved one if they cannot persuade him or her to engage in therapy. The best course of action in this case is to make sure they understand what therapy entails and the likely benefits. They may then decide not to engage in therapy at the current time. Throughout the years, I have seen many people who did not wish to engage in ERP when I first met them but, sometimes years later, came back and completed therapy and are now doing extremely well. In other words, the door should always be left open for the individual to accept ERP therapy in the future; it is never too late, and it is the individual with OCD who must decide when the time is right for them. On the other hand, some people have therapy and then wish to have more and more. ERP works by the person with OCD eventually learning to be their own therapist. If the individual has had a reasonable trial of therapy of approximately 20–40 sessions, then there should be a gap of six months to one year before any more therapy is prescribed. It is counterproductive to become fixated or 'addicted' to the therapy! A gap in therapy allows the individual to think about their goals of therapy and how best to apply ERP and to try to implement some of this themselves.

Another important reason for ERP not being successful is that it is not prescribed or performed in a regular, prolonged, predictable manner. For the best results, ERP should be practiced three times a day and for sufficient time to allow the anxiety to reduce consistently by at least 50 per cent.

Sometimes the wrong programmes are being applied. For example, someone may be performing ERP in the clinic but not be able to continue it at home. In such cases, it can be useful to return to easier items on the hierarchy and determine if they can then perform these at home. In other cases, it may be helpful for the therapist to go with the person to perform ERP in the home setting or wherever the symptoms are maximal.

Another issue arises when there is confusion over fear-provoking obsessions and anxiety-reducing compulsions. Exposure should be performed without the compulsions because the compulsions essentially neutralise the effect of exposure.

It can often be tempting to gradually reduce compulsions or even place these on a hierarchy. In reality, this rarely works because it is extremely difficult to cut down on such behaviours. It is much better and easier in the long term to stop the compulsive behaviours entirely. In the case of washing compulsion or other compulsions which are also necessary behaviours, the compulsive activity should be stopped and a new form of more 'normal' behaviour introduced and practiced.

Sometimes anxiety does not reduce after exposure due to certain medications or even alcohol. Tablets such as lorazepam (Ativan), diazepam (Valium), and chlordiazepoxide (Librium) are sometimes prescribed for people with OCD even though these should only be used for short periods of time up to a maximum of six weeks. It can be tempting for the individual who is feeling anxious to take one of these tablets. In such cases, the tablet taking is replacing the compulsions and will not result in a long-term reduction in anxiety. A similar action is found with alcohol, which can also be used in this manner.

Another reason why ERP may not work is that the person has a complicating additional diagnosis. Most people with moderate to severe OCD are also depressed. For the majority of people, treatment of the OCD also lifts the depression. This is not true, however, for a minority of people. Possible approaches to this are discussed in Chapter 6.

Similarly, some people have extremely high levels of anxiety and/or believe in the rationality of the obsessive thoughts. These cases, along with cases in which people have developed OCD following childhood trauma, are discussed in Chapter 6.

Finally, some people have problems controlling and tolerating their emotions. These people can find it almost impossible to engage with ERP. These individuals often have had a disrupted childhood and may be diagnosed with emotionally unstable personality disorder. It is often advisable for these people to receive help in learning how to tolerate strong emotions before embarking on ERP treatment.

Cognitive Therapy and OCD

Although it may seem logical to try to tackle OCD using cognitive therapy, there is no evidence that it offers any advantage compared to ERP. Many studies have been performed to examine any differences between the two approaches; overall, ERP generally produces similar or better results compared to any cognitive intervention. Indeed, any cognitive treatment requires an exposure element to be successful. Poorly applied cognitive therapy may make some patients with OCD worse. This is because the process of searching for evidence to confirm or refute the obsessions can become incorporated into the compulsive rituals. Cognitive therapy is also less cost-efficient because it requires more training and supervision for the therapist and usually takes more time to perform. Overall, this means that more people can be helped using ERP rather than cognitive behaviour therapy (CBT).

Probably the most logical usage of CBT is that the vast majority of people with OCD can be helped with the strategy of ERP, with or without medication. For people who cannot respond or who have an additional complicating diagnosis, specific CBT strategies may be used.

Other Forms of Psychological Treatment and OCD

There is no evidence that strategies such as counselling or psychotherapy which involve talking about the OCD problems are useful in the treatment of OCD. Indeed, in some cases these strategies may worsen the situation as the person becomes increasingly introspective.

Family therapy can sometimes be a useful addition to ERP treatment if the family are heavily involved in either helping the person with OCD perform their compulsions or if they are unduly negative towards the individual.

Key Points

- The exposure principle of treatment for OCD states that if the person exposes themselves to objects or situations which provoke the anxiety-provoking thoughts for a sufficient length of time (usually two hours) without performing anxiety-reducing compulsions, then their anxiety will reduce. This is known as exposure with self-imposed response prevention (ERP).

- ERP should be performed in a graded manner, starting with easier exposure items.

- ERP should be repeated regularly, ideally three times a day.

- Although anxiety is unpleasant, it will not lead to harm and will eventually reduce if no compulsions or avoidance behaviours are used.

- ERP can be applied to all types of OCD.

- ERP is successful in approximately 75 per cent of people who are offered the treatment.

- Sometimes ERP does not work because the individual is not yet ready to change and to give up their OCD.

- Other reasons why ERP may not work initially are that it is not being applied correctly or that a complicating additional diagnosis is preventing the anxiety from reducing.

- Cognitive behaviour therapy does not seem to add any benefit for most people with OCD above what can be achieved using ERP.

- Talking therapies in general are not helpful.

- Family therapy can be used in addition to ERP if there are specific family difficulties.

References

1. Drummond, L.M., and Fineberg, N.A (2007). Obsessive–compulsive disorders. In G. Stein, ed., *College Seminars in Adult Psychiatry*. London: Gaskell, pp. 270–86.

2. Exposure and self-imposed response prevention (ERP) adapted from Stern, R.S., and Drummond, L. M. (1991). *The Practice of Behavioural and Cognitive Psychotherapy*. Cambridge, UK: Cambridge University Press.

3. Tyagi, H., Drummond, L.M., and Fineberg, N.A. (2010). *Treatment for Obsessive Compulsive Disorder Current psychiatry Reviews*, 6(1), 46–55.

4. Boschen, M.J., Drummond, L.M., Pillay, A., and Morton, K. (2010). Predicting Outcome of Treatment for Severe, Treatment Resistant OCD in Inpatient and Community Settings. *Journal of Behavior Therapy and Experimental Psychiatry*, 41, 90–5.

Chapter

6

Children and Adolescents with OCD

This chapter will examine the recognition and treatment of children and adolescents with OCD. Until recently, OCD was thought to be rare in children. It is now recognized to be among the most common mental disorders in childhood. There are differences between the way OCD presents in childhood and that seen in adulthood. These differences are mainly due to children's lack of maturity. This chapter will give examples and pay particular attention to recognition using case examples. Treatment for children is similar to that for adults, but there are some clear differences. First, with very young children, it is difficult to set up a rigid hierarchy and expect them to learn to be their own therapist and so adaptation is necessary. Second, with young children, the entire family needs to be involved if the situation is not to unravel once treatment ends. Third, drug dosages are lower for children. Adolescents who present with OCD are often extremely dependent on their parents and have consequently had a very restrictive upbringing. These adolescents need help learning how to care for themselves and to engage with the world. Adolescence is a time of rebellion for many young people; for some, this means they will rebel against their treatment and fail to engage fully. Tips are given as to how to engage this group.

Finally, we will explore the idea of OCD arising acutely in childhood in some children and the possible relationship between this condition and infection. The controversial paediatric autoimmune neuropsychiatric disorders associated with streptococcal infection (PANDAS) or, more recently, paediatric/childhood acute-onset neuropsychiatric syndrome (PANS/CANS) will be discussed. These are based on the theory that some children have a very dramatic and sudden onset of OCD symptoms together with other neurological symptoms, such as extreme jerking, twitching, and loss of balance. The theory is that certain bacterial infections can trick the body to 'mistake' its own cells as being those of bacteria. In susceptible individuals, this may cause the body to attack its own cells in the brain. In a small minority of people with OCD, there is evidence that some cells in the basal ganglia (back of the brain) have been damaged in this manner. This has led to studies on the use of antibiotics in some children in the acute phase of onset.

OCD is one of the most common psychological problems seen in childhood. Whereas it was once thought to be rare in this age group, it is now known to be quite common, with between 1 and 3 per cent of children being affected. A recent large cross-national study of adults found that almost one in five adults with OCD gave a history of the condition starting before the age of ten years [1]. Fortunately, childhood OCD does not necessarily continue into adulthood. OCD can be extremely difficult to diagnose in young children for two main reasons. First, young children may not be able to express their thoughts and emotions in a coherent manner or may try to hide the behaviours from others. It has been suggested that it is almost impossible to diagnose OCD in children younger than age seven years. Second, children often experience periods in which they may have obsessive symptoms which resolve spontaneously.

Case Study 6.1

Bryony is a nine-year-old girl who is doing well in school, has friends, and generally appears to be a happy and healthy child. Six months ago, she was attending a local Brownie Guide meeting and discussion was held about the importance of hand hygiene. The children were shown pictures of the various types of bacteria. Bryony was very keen on watching medical dramas on television and said she wished to work in a hospital when she grew up. She was fascinated by watching the surgical staff 'scrub up' before performing operations. She started to perform the same type of washing before every meal, coming to the table with her hands in the air and wishing to repeat the wash if anyone contaminated her. Her mother had a long discussion with her and explained the reasons why this was not necessary. Bryony believed that bacteria were 'disgusting', but her mother encouraged her to also think of all the good things bacteria are capable of doing. After a few weeks, this behaviour completely subsided because Bryony found it was too time-consuming to continue, and she developed an interest in learning more about the ways in which bacteria can protect against allergies.

This story shows how, with the family treating her concerns as a normal phase of development and not taking them too seriously, the 'phase' passed and Bryony was left with no residual symptoms. Not every situation is similar, however, and it can be difficult to diagnose the disorder in children if the content of the obsessive thoughts and compulsive rituals changes over time.

Case Study 6.2

George is an 11-year-old boy who was first noted by his parents at age eight years to be acting strangely. He would scream and become distressed if any mud landed on him or his clothing. Not wanting to play in the park, George started to complain that he had tummy pain on the days at school when students were due to play football or other outside sports. Believing this to 'be a phase', his parents asked the school to excuse him from sports. However, this extreme avoidance of mud led him to be teased and bullied at school. Suddenly, the problem seemed to stop and he returned to playing outside again. However, his parents noticed that he would periodically stand still and blow into the air. This would last several minutes. At the same time, his school performance started to suffer, and he began to get into trouble at school for failing to hand in his work on time. His parents became worried and took George to see his general practitioner, who referred him to the local child and adolescent mental health service. Initially, it was difficult to find out from George what was bothering him. The family were seen together, and it was decided to also see George alone. After several sessions with the therapist, George admitted that he had extreme worries that his parents might die. These could occur at any time of the day or night, but when he had the thoughts, he had the urge to stand completely still and 'blow the thoughts away'. Unbeknown to his parents, George was waking up several times at night and quietly entering their bedroom to ensure he could still hear them breathing. This meant he was getting little sleep, and so his school performance was deteriorating.

Treatment for George consisted of a meeting with all the family to discuss the OCD – what it is and how it can be treated. George is an only child, and at the time he was very worried that his parents were older than most and so might die sooner, leaving him alone. Exposure and response prevention (ERP) consisted of George being encouraged to bring on his obsessive thoughts without performing the compulsions of repeated checking and blowing. This was extremely stressful, and he became very distressed and unable to continue. In light of this, it was decided to introduce additional treatment with sertraline. The dose of sertraline was adjusted to take into account George's age and size. He was started on a low dose of 25 mg, and this was gradually increased every week until he was on half the normal adult dose.

Once on sertraline, George appeared much brighter and was better able to engage with the ERP programme. He is currently doing well and is looking forward to moving to senior school next summer.

What Differences Need to Be Applied for Children in the ERP Programme?

Treatment of children who have OCD with ERP is identical to that for adults, except it is unreasonable to expect young children to learn the principles of the therapy and apply it themselves. For this reason, the family should normally be actively involved. Understanding OCD and the negative effect that compulsive rituals and reassurance-seeking can have on the condition is an important part of the discussion. It can be very difficult for a parent to resist offering reassurance to their distressed child and so there needs to be a frank and full discussion in terms that the child can understand. Making a statement such as 'Mummy loves you very much and for that reason I am not going to answer your question. You remember how we talked about how answering these questions make you more anxious?' can be helpful. It can seem to the child that a parent is being deliberatively punitive if they do refuse to answer, and so a reminder of previous discussions can be helpful. However, children are very good at 'holding their parents to ransom', and if it is late at night and everyone is tired and wants to go to bed, it can seem impossible not to give the reassurance that is required. If this happens, it is not a disaster. (It can be helpful for children to see that their parents are 'fallible'!) Of importance is that the child understands that they are loved but that part of this love is that the parent will no longer give reassurance because this will only end up making the situation worse.

In addition, with young children it is sometimes important that the whole family be involved in treatment.

Case Study 6.3

Mari is an active eight-year-old who lives with her mother and two older siblings. A year after her father left the family home when Mari was six years old, her mother moved the family to a new house that was much larger than the old one and also had white carpets and new furniture. Six months ago, Mari began to be overly concerned about keeping her room and the house tidy and was constantly worried that she may make a mess. Mari's mother worried that she had nagged the children too much about making a mess and that this had caused Mari's problem. Due to her feelings of guilt, she would reassure Mari constantly. Treatment involved all the family deliberately leaving some of the rooms untidy. When Mari asked for reassurance about being tidy, her mother told her that she did not mind whether the house was 'messy' or not. One final exposure programme involved all the family having a picnic in the living room on the white carpet. When they had finished, they all rolled around on the floor and ended up having a boisterous game with much laughing. Mari is now a much happier and relaxed child who is enjoying school and home life. Her mother reports that 'everyone is much happier now that I am more relaxed about the house. I have realised it is more important to have a happy rather than a perfect home'.

In the story of Mari, the entire family was able to relax and gain a better perspective and a calmer attitude towards life due to the ERP treatment. This does not mean that everyone should live in chaos and mess but, rather, that it is worthwhile to think about achieving a balance where everyone can be happy. Mari's mother also worried that she had 'caused' her daughter's OCD. In general, it is neither helpful nor possible to apportion blame in this way. Mari had experienced a number of changes in her life which may or may not have been related to the onset of her disorder. Some children with normal lives and little upset can develop OCD symptoms, whereas others who experience extreme trauma may be fine and may not develop problems. The important point in this case is that the entire family is now more settled and happy with their current situation, and there is every hope that Mari will continue to have a happy and healthy childhood.

Surely If a Child Has OCD It Is Due to Bad Parenting or to Upsetting Incidents?

The story of Mari illustrates how it is very easy for parents to blame themselves for their children's problems. The situation, however, is far more complicated than this.

We know that OCD has a tendency to run in families. Therefore, if a close family member has OCD, there is a greater chance that the children may also develop it. Again, this is far from inevitable, and more children will not develop OCD than those who do. Because people see some similarities in the behaviour of both the parent and the child in situations in which both have OCD, there is a tendency for people to blame the parent for 'causing' the condition. This is unfair. The parent can no more be held responsible for having OCD or OC traits to their personality than can the child. Both have been dealt a genetic predisposition to develop OCD just as a parent cannot be blamed for their child having blond hair or blue eyes. In Chapter 2, we discussed resilience, which appears to be partly inherited and partly influenced by a warm, happy home environment. Despite this idea of resilience, some children brought up in a warm, loving home will still develop OCD. In other words, it is pointless to lay the blame at anyone's feet for a child developing OCD. It is much more important to seek help and to start the child on the path to a happy and healthy future.

Many researchers have examined whether disruption in a child's life results in OCD. There is no conclusive evidence on this issue, with some studies linking OCD to previous life events in childhood and some finding no association.

Drug Treatment for OCD in Childhood

Most children with OCD will respond to ERP treatment and will not require drug treatment. Some children, however, will need to have a trial of medication as well.

The drug treatment of choice for children with OCD is the use of selective serotonin reuptake inhibitors (SSRIs) (see Chapter 4). The doses used in children are smaller than those used in adults and are related to children's smaller size (Table 6.1). Generally, drugs for children should be prescribed according to their weight.

Clomipramine is also sometimes prescribed to children. The reservations expressed in Chapter 4 also apply to children. Because clomipramine tends to have a greater risk of side effects compared to SSRIs, it should not be used as a first-line treatment. It should be introduced at a low dose starting at 10 mg/day

Table 6.1 Drugs which are commonly used for OCD in children in the United Kingdom

Drug	Trade name	Dose range used in children (increasing with age up to ten years)
Fluoxetine	Prozac	20–60 mg/day The average is 1 mg per kilogram body weight per day. For example, a 40-kg child would be prescribed 40 mg/day.
Sertraline	Lustral	25–200 mg/day Generally start at 25 mg/day and increase after one week to 50 mg/day. Any further increase depends on the age and weight of the child.
Paroxetine	Seroxat	10–60 mg/day
Fluvoxamine	Faverin	100–250 mg/day
Citalopram	Cipramil	10–40 mg/day Can increase by 5 mg per day every two weeks depending on the age and weight of the child.

and should be gradually increased to a maximum of 3 mg/kg/day or 200 mg/day (whichever is less). Clomipramine is not recommended for children younger than age ten years.

If the child has not responded to cognitive behaviour therapy involving ERP and a trial of two different SSRIs for a minimum of three months each, more specialised help is needed. Other drugs, such as dopamine blockers, can be added into the regimen, but particular care needs to be taken in using them in young people, who are more prone to side effects.

It is known that people who respond to SSRIs often relapse when these drugs are stopped. After approximately a year of treatment, it may be possible to reduce or stop the SSRI treatment. This should be done gradually and under the supervision of a health care professional. The main risks are withdrawal side effects as well as a relapse of OCD.

People are often reluctant to allow their children to take SSRIs. It should be remembered that these drugs are not used to 'numb' or 'sedate' the child but, rather, are prescribed to try to increase the amount of serotonin in the brain, which is at a low level due to OCD.

Adolescents with OCD

Adolescence is often a tricky time. Teenagers often appear grumpy, aloof from their family, and secretive but impulsive, and they can rapidly switch from being fiercely independent to behaving like a child again. These are all a normal part of this stage of development into adulthood as young people try to establish in their own minds who they are and what they want. This inevitably means trying to separate themselves from the family as they strive to assert their independence. In addition, adolescence is a time of changes in hormones and discovery of sexuality, along with feelings of self-doubt about appearance and attractiveness.

For a young person who also has OCD, adolescence is particularly difficult. They may struggle with wanting to go out and do the things that their friends are doing but find that their OCD prevents them from doing so. OCD often causes them to be more dependent and more in the position of a much younger child. Indeed, the fact that OCD can prevent this natural separation, individuation, and maturation from happening means that young people with OCD, even those who are well into young adulthood, can appear much younger than their years, regardless of how intellectually able they may be. In addition, normal sexual thoughts, impulses, and experimentation may be a source of huge guilt to the young person with OCD.

Those who develop OCD in adolescence might not discuss the disorder with their parents or people in authority. Adolescents very often try to hide their problems and sort them out themselves. It can be particularly difficult for parents to become aware of OCD problems because 'normal' adolescents often spend increasing amounts of time alone in their rooms and prolonged time in the bathroom as they try to come to terms with their own image as a sexually-attractive adult. For parents of adolescents, the key is to leave the lines of communication between parent and offspring as open as possible. This means not talking 'down' to them but, rather, being open and honest about issues. Young people dislike being 'preached' at or 'nagged', and it is often a juggling act for a parent to maintain interest in their son or daughter without appearing overly intrusive and overbearing. Often, the young person is more relaxed in situations away from home and where they do not feel 'trapped' by the parent. The parent has to learn to listen more than they talk to the adolescent. This can be difficult to do. With younger children, the parental role is more about advice and guidance, whereas with adolescents the parent has to withdraw slightly and trust that the early lessons they have instilled in their child will stand the adolescent in good stead. While the parent is driving, for example, can be a time that the young person feels more able to talk, without direct eye contact and when the parent is preoccupied with another task and so will not react as strongly to whatever is said.

Signs that a young person may have problems with OCD, apart from clear and obvious excessive washing for no reason and checking compulsions, include the following:

- An unexpected poor performance at school
- Unauthorised absence from school
- Spending hours in the bathroom and/or toilet
- Appearing distracted
- Losing friends or struggling to make friends
- Worries that occur repeatedly
- Distress when a compulsive action is interrupted
- Getting in trouble at school for slowness or compulsions

None of these signs is exclusive to OCD. Most are seen in a range of psychological disorders as well as normal adolescence, but it is the combination of these signs together with information that can be gleaned from the adolescents themselves which may point to OCD being a problem.

Although adolescents need a degree of freedom and autonomy, they also need firm boundaries which are adhered to. These boundaries clearly need to be more liberal than with a younger child, but they still need to exist. Young people will often rebel against these boundaries, their parents, those in authority, and the system in which they live. For a young person with OCD, this can often take the form of rebelling against their treatment. Many young people with OCD who are up to 25 years of age will often rebel and refuse to participate in therapy, even though they wish to overcome their OCD. The thought of working with a structured therapy is just too overwhelming. In such cases, it is often useful to ask them what they would like their life to be like in one or two years. Where would they be living? What job/type of study would they be doing? What would their social life be like? From this, it can be determined with them what they are currently able to do. Then it must be worked out with them what skills they need to develop and what tasks they need to conquer to start edging towards their dreams. Adolescents often respond better to this type of approach rather than to a structured ERP regime. In reality, the end result is the same because by developing their skills, they generally need to perform ERP as well. The more 'problem-solving' approach can be better tolerated by some adolescents.

PANDAs, PANs, and CANs

In recent years, there has been interest in and research on the idea that an infection may be involved in a proportion of children or adolescents with OCD. An extremely small proportion of children and adolescents seem to develop symptoms of OCD with an extremely rapid onset. This occurs in only 1 in 20 children with OCD. In these situations, the OCD is often accompanied by abnormal movements or sudden loss of coordination. These children sometimes have physical symptoms similar to those seen in a tiny proportion of children after a specific form of bacterial throat infection. The vast majority of throat infections are caused by viruses, and they cause no long-term problems. Some more severe throat infections are caused by a specific bacterium known as beta-haemolytic streptococcus group A (strep). Some weeks after a strep sore throat, susceptible individuals have been known to present with

- abnormal movements (sometimes known as Sydenham's chorea/St Vitus dance); and
- problems with the heart and painful joints (rheumatic fever).

These problems are thought to occur as a result of an autoimmune response whereby the body tries to fight the infection. In certain susceptible individuals, the body not only 'attacks' the strep infection but also mistakenly attacks some of its own cells. In rheumatic fever, it attacks some cells in the joints and the heart, and in chorea it attacks some brain cells. Children who have such problems do get better, but there can also be long-term damage. There has been a very marked reduction in these complications of strep infections in developed countries since the early twentieth century. The reason for this reduction is not well understood, but it is thought to be due to the availability of antibiotics and the better general health and nutrition of children in the Western world. Skin rashes (scarlet fever) can also follow a strep sore throat after just a few days, but unlike the other conditions, these rashes occur earlier and are highly infectious, and they are not related to the same autoimmune diseases.

PANDAS is still a controversial concept, and not all child mental health workers are convinced it exists. It has been more widely accepted in the United States than in Europe. The condition can present with an extremely rapid onset of abnormal movements associated with tics, Tourette's syndrome, or OCD. In those with OCD, it appears that the symptoms generally improve over weeks or months. The children are particularly susceptible to side effects of SSRIs, and so these need to be used with care. It appears that the part of the brain known as the basal ganglia (the same area where the dopamine blockers act) is attacked by antibodies. If a child is suspected to have PANDAS, it is important to treat future sore throat episodes rapidly with antibiotics. Once the symptoms have presented, antibiotics are unlikely to give much benefit.

More recently, it has become clear that strep is not the only infection which can appear to precipitate tics or OCD in susceptible individuals. For this reason, it has been suggested that the term be altered to either PANS or CANS.

It is important to remember that the number of children affected by this type of problem is extremely small. Most children catch all kinds of infections without problems or, indeed, with the benefit of building their immunity. Thus, although interesting, in most situations OCD appears to be unrelated to infections, but future research of this type may help us better understand the development of OCD.

In reality, most children with OCD, even those with acute onset of OCD, will respond to treatment with ERP. Drug treatment may have to be used carefully because there is a suggestion that some children with this type of OCD are more likely to experience side effects. Antibiotics are only useful if the child is still showing signs of infection.

Key Points

- Once thought to be rare in childhood, OCD is now known to be relatively common, affecting 1–3 per cent of children.
- OCD in childhood is similar to that seen in adults but can be difficult to diagnose due to children's lack of maturity and inability to explain their difficulties.

- ERP treatment may need to be adapted for younger patients, and family involvement is important.

- OCD medication for children is identical to that prescribed for adults except that the dose prescribed will be lower depending on the young person's age, size, and weight.

- Adolescents may also present particular challenges where the OCD can be combined with the frequent rebellion of adolescence.

- PANDAS, PANS, or CANS is the rapid onset of OCD or a tic disorder, usually with a marked and obvious onset of a movement disorder, in a young person who has recently suffered from an infection. It is believed that the bacteria 'trick' the immune system into attacking the individual's own cells. These children usually respond to cognitive behaviour therapy.

Reference

1. Dell'oss B., Benatti B., Hollander E., et al. (2016) Childhood, adolescent and adult age at onset and related clinical correlates in obsessive-compulsive disorder: a report from the International College of Obsessive-Compulsive Spectrum Disorders (ICOCS). *International Journal of Psychiatry in Clinical Practice*, 20(4) 210–17.

Chapter

Old Treatments, Modern Developments, New Research, and Potential Treatments for the Future

This chapter will examine ongoing research and the potential role this may have in the future. The chapter will first discuss physical methods of treatment. Then it will examine the role of infection and inflammation in the development of OCD. Finally, it examines potential gene modification by some hormones and how these may be harnessed to improve the outcome in OCD in the future.

First, there will be an examination of the role that neurosurgery has played for a very small number of people with OCD who have failed to respond to all other treatment approaches. This will dispel the myth that neurosurgery is the same as the 'lobotomy' performed during the early twentieth century. The reported outcomes of more specific surgery performed today will also be examined.

The chapter then discusses recent research into deep brain stimulation for people who may previously have been sent for neurosurgery. This technique still involves wires being placed in the brain, but it does not permanently destroy brain tissue in the way neurosurgery does.

Next, the chapter will examine the more experimental transcranial magnetic stimulation as a potential alternative to more invasive procedures and possibly a technique which may be used in more routine practice in the future. This technique involves the application of powerful magnets to the outside of the head. By targeting these to act on specific areas on the brain, they can temporarily reduce OCD symptomatology. It is hoped that these may be useful in combination with exposure and response prevention (ERP) for some people unable to tolerate ERP alone.

In another area of research, it has been suggested that the glial cells in the brains of people with autism and OCD may be inflamed and unable to act normally. These cells produce glutamate, and this may tie in with recent work examining the potential use of glutamate modifiers. This theory has been taken further by some, who theorize that the normal healthy bacteria which make up an important part of our bodies may have become altered in modern life, resulting in an increase in autoimmune conditions. It has been suggested that childhood autism may also be 'autoimmune'. People with autism often have marked OCD symptoms, and so this link is also being examined.

Finally, the chapter will discuss how certain hormones may modify our genes. We know that OCD is a condition with a complex causation. Although there seems to be a genetic link, there is no clear pattern of inheritance, suggesting that other factors may be acting in a 'preventative' way to prevent OCD from always appearing in its full-blown form. One theory is that oxytocin, a hormone produced when one is being nurtured or is nurturing, may bind to the gene and make it more likely to be dormant. Thus, it might be possible that good nurturing experiences in early childhood may modify or reduce OCD symptoms for some, but not all, people with OCD.

Brain Surgery

The whole concept of brain surgery is controversial and arouses strong opinions and emotions in some people [1]. Undoubtedly, the procedures of the past were brutal and resulted in massive side effects. It must be noted that until the mid-1950s, we did not have the powerful medications which could help many people without resorting to, what seems to us today, extreme measures. Today's interventions are far more targeted but still give rise to considerable controversy. In the United Kingdom today, we can assert with absolute confidence that no one would ever receive brain surgery for OCD in the National Health Service without first receiving all other available treatments and failing to improve with those and also without having been fully informed of all the potential risks and benefits and subsequently consenting to the procedures. Neurosurgery is a very rare procedure for OCD, generally because ERP and drug treatment tend to work extremely well for most people. Brain surgery is, and will remain, the last resort for a very few individuals who do not benefit from less invasive procedures.

Is Brain Surgery Like I Have Seen in Films?

There have been many depictions on stage and screen of brain surgery, and these generally paint a terrifying picture. In the early days of psychiatry, there were no effective drugs for psychological and psychiatric disorders. Most people with long-standing psychiatric problems were admitted to long-stay hospitals or asylums where they were kept apart from society and given food, nourishment, and a roof over their heads. Various 'treatments' which appear outlandish today were tried, including ice baths, insulin coma treatment, and sleep deprivation. Although these appear barbaric, it must be remembered that the lack of effective drugs or psychological therapies meant that there were no real therapeutic options and so people tried methods that they hoped would improve the plight of those admitted to asylums. The 'treatment' of prefrontal leucotomy was introduced in the 1930s and was performed via two small holes in the head through which a sharp instrument was introduced which removed the connections between frontal parts and the bulk of the brain. This was introduced not as a direct treatment for mental disorder but, rather, as a way of inducing calm in the individual. This procedure was performed on hundreds of patients throughout the world before being replaced by a similar procedure which was just as crude, called prefrontal lobotomy. This procedure involved sharp implements going through the back of the eye sockets to achieve the same aim. It was developed by neurologists, Dr Freeman and Dr Watts, and because it could be performed easily, Dr Freeman claimed to have personally overseen up to 3,500 operations by the 1960s. In the mid-1950s, due to the development of both antipsychotic and antidepressant drugs, the demand for these surgical procedures rapidly declined. There was a significant mortality rate associated with the procedures. In addition, they were applied to any individual who was highly agitated and thus were used for people with schizophrenia, depression, and anxiety disorders as well as OCD.

More Modern and Precise Surgery

During the 1970s and 1980s, there was better understanding of the functions of various parts of the brain and operations were developed, mostly for intractable depression and OCD, which caused much less widespread brain damage but aimed to target specific areas of the brain. For example, a group in South West London developed a procedure known as 'limbic leucotomy' which involved small incisions or lesions being made in an area in the front of the brain. This was reported for use in people with OCD who did not respond to other treatments. It was followed by intensive ERP treatment and appeared to show good results, with 84 per cent of people with OCD showing lasting benefit with few long-lasting side effects [2]. Overall, four types of neurosurgical operations which cause permanent lesions have been used for OCD:

- Limbic leucotomy
- Subcaudate tractotomy
- Cingulotomy
- Capsulotomy

These procedures all involve lesions within the frontal area of the brain. The widespread damage caused by earlier operations no longer occurs because of new ways in which surgeons can obtain images of the brains of individuals. Good outcomes have been reported for people with OCD. However, it must be remembered that none of these procedures have been fully investigated using the usual 'controlled trial' method of evaluation in which a 'dummy' or 'sham' procedure is compared with the treatment. This is because it is clearly unethical to submit a very unwell individual to a general anaesthetic and drill holes in the skull without performing a procedure. Currently, these procedures are limited in the United Kingdom to those who have failed to respond to repeated trials of both medication and ERP and who have profound OCD. Only a tiny handful of these operations are performed (less than one per year). The individual must always give informed consent, and there is also a legal procedure surrounding permission for surgery. These procedures depend on the country in which the person lives. In England and Wales, a second opinion appointed doctor (SOAD) and two other people appointed by the Care Quality Commission in England or the Healthcare Inspectorate Wales certify that the person has the capacity to consent and has done so. The SOAD also certifies that it is appropriate for a person to receive the treatment. In Scotland, a designated medical practitioner, appointed by the Mental Welfare Commission, has to provide an independent opinion that the procedure will be beneficial. Two laypeople appointed by the Commission must then certify whether or not the individual has the capacity to consent and has done so. Variations of these laws exist in other European countries, in Australasia, and in the United States and Canada.

Deep Brain Stimulation

A different approach to permanently destroying areas of brain tissue is the use of electrodes to stimulate differing areas of the brain to help overcome OCD symptoms. In this procedure, brain tissue is not destroyed, but electrical stimulation is used to alter the circuitry which results in OCD symptoms. This operation still requires a general anaesthetic. Small holes are then made in the skull through which thin wires are inserted and, using modern brain imaging techniques, these are moved to stimulate relevant areas in the front of the brain. A battery pack is then inserted in the chest wall to enable a small electrical current to provide electrical stimulation.

Deep brain stimulation (DBS) was first introduced as a highly successful treatment for the movement disorder Parkinson's disease. During approximately the past ten years, DBS has also been investigated for use in the treatment of severe depression, Tourette's syndrome, and OCD. There have been a number of studies of DBS in OCD, but various different areas in the pathways have been stimulated, and it is sometimes difficult to compare outcomes. A study of all cases of DBS used for OCD which were reported in the medical literature from 1999 to 2014 showed that there were a total of 31 studies involving 116 people. Overall, a 45 per cent reduction in symptoms was reported by the participants. Sixty per cent of people responded to the treatment. Various different targets were used for stimulation in the studies [3].

A recent study in the United Kingdom examined people who had failed all other treatments and who were being considered for neurosurgery. Six people received DBS in up to four stimulation areas, and these were all compared until the best setting for each individual was found. All six patients showed marked improvements in their OCD symptoms, with more than a 35 per cent reduction in symptoms [4].

Overall, DBS seems to be a promising treatment for those who have the most profound OCD which does not respond to all other drug and ERP treatments.

Are There Any New and Less Invasive Treatments for People Who Do Not Respond to Drug Therapy and ERP?

A new and novel possibility is the use of transcranial magnetic stimulation (TMS). This involves applying powerful magnets to the outside of the skull. By directing these appropriately, it is possible to reduce activity in specific areas of the brain on a temporary basis. Often, this is repeated on a regular basis. Regular TMS has been shown to be useful in treating some people with severe migraine and also depression. For depression, TMS is applied daily for a period of up to six weeks.

There is evidence that TMS can improve symptoms for people with OCD which does not respond to other treatments [5]. However, there are many different approaches to this treatment. For treatment of OCD, the magnets used with TMS must be more powerful than those used for depression to penetrate deeper into the brain. Also, this treatment must be repeated regularly, but it is unclear how long it should be repeated for it to have a lasting benefit.

One of the differences between OCD and depression is that bouts of depression often last a few months at a time and are interspersed by periods of feeling well, whereas OCD is often, but not always, a consistent and continuous condition. It may therefore be problematic if a shorter treatment regimen is used. Research is needed to examine not only the efficacy but also the optimal way to deliver TMS to people with OCD. Furthermore, the combination of TMS with ERP is worthy of further study.

Inflammation and OCD

In Chapter 6, we discussed the way in which it appears that certain bacteria can trick the body into producing antibodies which then attack certain parts of the body instead of attacking the bacteria. These are known to cause autoimmune disorders, including conditions such as rheumatoid arthritis, coeliac disease, childhood-onset diabetes, psoriasis, and asthma. It may be that autoimmunity is implicated in a small proportion of children who develop rapid-onset movement disorders and OCD.

Another recent theory is that inflammation of the glial cells in the brain can give rise to childhood autism and possibly OCD [6]. The work has generally been based on children with autism who also often have OCD symptoms. It has been shown that in some individuals with these conditions, the glial cells of the brain are inflamed. Glial cells were discussed in Chapter 4. These are the cells which occupy spaces between the neurones, which are the cells that transmit messages through the brain. The glial cells' function seems to be to modulate and control the transmission of messages. Glutamate is the chemical which is released by the glial cells, and it plays a role in helping control this transmission. In Chapter 4, we discussed drugs which act on the glutamate system and appear to make OCD worse or better. Some researchers have suggested that the inflammation of the glial cells upsets glutamate secretion results in the OCD symptoms of autism.

These researchers also suggest that autoimmune conditions are increasing in modern society. This increase is suggested to be related to the overly clean and hygienic conditions in which children are raised. Whereas in the past, young children were exposed to a wider variety of bacteria and their immune systems learned to cope with them at a very young age, in modern society children are often kept in extremely clean environments during their very early years. This may mean that their bodies do not know how to cope with the range of bacteria they encounter later on in childhood, making them more prone to autoimmune disease. Indeed, recent research suggests that children who grow up on farms and who are exposed to a range of bacteria from a variety of animals are much less likely to develop asthma [7]. Some researchers suggest that the restriction of bacteria in the gut, by living in ultra-clean environments and by the use of antibiotics, may lead to the development of OCD in susceptible individuals. These researchers believe that changes in the bacteria in the gut are the reason why OCD often develops during pregnancy (when hormonal changes affect the gut bacteria) or following a strep sore throat (due to treatment with antibiotics upsetting the gut bacteria) [8]. These theories are far from proven and are all highly speculative, but they do raise some interesting questions about our modern environment and the possible development of new treatments for OCD.

Can Genes Be Modified? What Is Oxytocin?

We have already examined how although OCD tends to run in families and to have a genetic basis, this is not the whole story. Having a parent, or even two parents or close relatives, with OCD does not necessarily mean that the child will develop OCD. In Chapter 2, we examined how early life experience may modify the genetic predisposition and lead to increased resilience. Resilience to life events may be partly inherited but may also be increased by the experience of a calm, loving, stable home environment. This does not mean that some people who have had a good home life and early life experience will not develop OCD, just that such an environment may modify the risk in those with a genetic predisposition to develop OCD. If early life experience can have an effect on resilience, how does this happen? One of many theories is that this may be related to oxytocin.

Oxytocin is a hormone which is produced by the brain in an area known as the hypothalamus. This hormone is sometimes called the 'love' hormone because it is the chemical which is produced when a mother suckles her baby, when a child or adult is being cuddled, or when we stare into the eyes of our loved one. It is thus a hormone which seems to induce caring and nurturing. It has been suggested that oxytocin may be the substance which binds to the affected genes in OCD and makes them less likely to be active. This is highly speculative and has not been fully tested.

It has also been noted that people with OCD have high levels of oxytocin in their blood and also in their brains. This has led some researchers to suggest that they may be causative in some way. High levels of oxytocin in blood seem to be correlated with more severe OCD symptoms. When given selective serotonin reuptake inhibitor or clomipramine treatment, individuals who respond show an initial decrease in oxytocin levels followed by an increase. Those who do not respond to drug treatment seem to show the opposite [9].

In summary, it is known that oxytocin levels are high in people with OCD. Whether this finding has any bearing on the development of OCD and whether it can be used to develop new treatments are yet to be explored.

Key Points

- In the nineteenth and early twentieth centuries, surgical procedures for psychiatric conditions including OCD were crude and had high rates of mortality and morbidity.

- Modified surgical procedures developed in the 1970s and 1980s are more specific, cause less brain damage, and have a lower risk. Studies suggest that these procedures are effective in most people who undergo them. No controlled trials have been performed.

- Deep brain stimulation (DBS) is another surgical procedure which does not cause permanent brain damage. Various sites in the brain have been investigated and have produced variable results. Overall, approximately 60 per cent of people with OCD who have previously failed to respond to other treatments improve significantly with DBS.

- Transcranial magnetic stimulation is another approach. This does not involve a surgical procedure. Powerful magnets are applied outside the skull and then temporarily interrupt the brain circuits causing OCD symptoms. This approach is still under investigation with regard to its possible role in the management of OCD.

- More speculative theories were discussed:

    · The possible role of inflammation of the glial cells was explored. Theories linking this and OCD to autoimmunity were also mentioned, as was the possible effect of gut bacteria on autoimmunity.

    · The role of oxytocin in protecting against OCD and the altered patterns of secretion in OCD were also discussed.

References

1. Heller, A. C., Amar, A. P., Liu, C. Y., and Apuzzo, M. L. (2006). Surgery of the Mind and Mood: A Mosaic of Issues in Time and Evolution. *Neurosurgery*, 59(4), 720–33; discussion 733–9.

2. Mitchell-Heggs, N., Kelly, D., and Richardson, A. (1976). Stereotactic Limbic Leucotomy – A Follow-up at 16 Months. *British Journal of Psychiatry*, 128, 126.

3. Alonso, P., Cuadras, D., Gabriëls, L., et al.(2015). Deep Brain Stimulation for Obsessive-Compulsive Disorder: A Meta-Analysis of Treatment Outcome and Predictors of Response. *PLoS One*, 10(7), e0133591.

4. Tyagi, H., Zrinzo, L., Foltynie, T., et al. (2016). Deep Brain Stimulation for Severe Obsessive-Compulsive Disorder. International Congress of the Royal College of Psychiatrists, *EXCEL, London*, 27–30 June.

5. Trevizol, A. P., Shiozawa, P., Cook, I. A. et al. (2016). Transcranial Magnetic Stimulation for Obsessive-Compulsive Disorder: An Updated Systematic Review and Meta-analysis, *The Journal of ECT*, 32(4):262–6.

6. Uzunova, G., Hollander, E., and Shepherd, J. (2014). The Role of Ionotropic Glutamate Receptors in Childhood Neurodevelopmental Disorders: Autism Spectrum Disorders and Fragile X Syndrome. *Current Neuropharmacology*, 12(1), 71–98. doi: 10.2174/1570159X113116660046

7. Birzele, L. T., Depner, M., Ege, M. J. et al. (2017). Environmental and Mucosal Microbiota and Their Role in Childhood Asthma. *Allergy*, 72(1), 109–19.

8. Rees, J. C. (2014). Obsessive–Compulsive Disorder and Gut Microbiota Dysregulation. *Medical Hypotheses*, 82(2), 163–6. doi: 10.1016/j.mehy.2013.11.026

9. Humble, M. B., Uvnäs-Moberg, K., Engström, I., and Bejerot, S. (2013). Plasma Oxytocin Changes and Anti-Obsessive Response during Serotonin Reuptake Inhibitor Treatment: A Placebo Controlled Study. *BMC Psychiatry*, 13, 344. doi: 10.1186/1471-244X-13-344

Chapter

8

Other Conditions Which Appear Similar to OCD

This chapter will examine a range of conditions which are often mistaken for OCD and which have similarities with OCD. There will be a brief mention of how these can be treated, and the evidence for both drug therapies and cognitive behaviour therapy (CBT) is also discussed. Case history illustrations are presented. The conditions covered will include the following:

- *Body dysmorphic disorder* (BDD): This section on BDD will examine the similarities between OCD and BDD, but also some of the differences. It will also examine the evidence for drug treatment and how the evidence suggests that higher dosages of selective serotonin reuptake inhibitors (SSRIs) are more likely to be needed in BDD. CBT treatment usually involves exposure and response prevention (ERP), but there is also usually a greater need to examine some of the underlying beliefs and the causes of low self-esteem, which is common in people with BDD.

- *Hoarding disorder*: There has been relatively little research into the area of hoarding disorder because this condition has only recently been recognised and come to prominence. Compared to people with OCD, people with hoarding disorder are more likely to be older and to be living alone. Although little is known about hoarding disorder, research suggests that some drugs may be useful, as might CBT aimed at helping the individual to stop acquiring new items whilst discarding old items.

- *Tourette's syndrome*: This condition is often accompanied by OCD symptoms. We will explore what this syndrome is and how it may be treated.

- *Hair pulling* (trichotillomania): This is a condition which has only recently been recognised as a separate psychiatric condition. There is a general lack of research in this area. Current treatment will be discussed.

- *Skin picking*: Again, this is a condition with little general recognition and little research. The severity of this condition can range from trivial to devastating and even life-endangering. Current research and treatment will be discussed.

- *Health anxiety*: Health anxiety has many similarities to OCD. There are intrusive, unwanted, worrying thoughts that the person has a serious disease. This worry causes high anxiety, and the person tries to abate this by performing a number of checks on themselves, by researching the Internet repeatedly, or by seeking reassurance from medical personal or friends and family. Repeated trips to medical facilities can sometimes result in extreme and excessive investigation with little evidence to support any serious physical pathology.

The fifth edition of the *Diagnostic and Statistical Manual of Mental Disorders* (DSM-5) is used widely throughout the world for classification of diseases and also for research [1]. If a disorder is not listed in the manual, there is likely to be much less research and study on the condition. In Europe and many other countries, a different but similar type of manual is used which is produced by the World Health Organisation. The *International Classification of Diseases* (ICD) covers all diseases and disorders, including those associated with mental health [2]. Currently, there are plans to update the ICD, which was published in 2004, and it is likely to follow a similar line as DSM-5 with respect to obsessive compulsive and related disorders.

Compared to previous versions, the DSM-5 had a number of significant changes regarding OCD and related conditions. Notably, OCD was removed from the section for anxiety disorders and placed in its own individual category of obsessive–compulsive and related disorders (Table 8.1).

It is recognised that tic disorder, most notably Tourette's syndrome, is often associated with OCD, but this is placed in the neuropsychiatric category in the DSM-5 due to the overlap of neurology and psychiatry in this condition. Another condition with many similarities to OCD, health anxiety, is included under a different classification of somatoform disorders. Both of these conditions will be discussed later.

Body Dysmorphic Disorder

Body dysmorphic disorder has many similarities to OCD. Until the 1990s, it was often either treated as OCD or, in more severe cases, considered an example of a psychotic disorder with one main symptom. In BDD, there is a preoccupation that a specific part of the body is ugly, deformed, or abnormal in some way. These thoughts cause distress, anxiety, and discomfort. In order to try to reduce these thoughts and feelings, the person with BDD may avoid a number of situations. In the most extreme cases, people with BDD may not leave their home at all or only do so under the cover of darkness. Some people will wear clothing, makeup, and accessories to try to reduce the exposure of the feature they dislike. This can often backfire, as it did with Siobhan.

Table 8.1 Disorders which have been included in the category of obsessive–compulsive and related disorders

Condition	What is it?	What are the main treatments?	Other points of interest
Body dysmorphic disorder (BDD)	This condition has many similarities to OCD, but the individual is preoccupied by what they believe is a major physical defect in their appearance.	Treatments involve CBT including exposure and response prevention combined with some cognitive therapy to examine some of the core beliefs about their perceived 'abnormalities'.\n\nDrug treatment with SSRI drugs or clomipramine has been demonstrated to be useful.	Many people with BDD also have social anxiety.
Hoarding disorder	Although some people with OCD also hoard items due to fear of disposing of items as a result of an obsessive fear such as fear of contamination or fear of loss of objects/information. In hoarding disorder, this is different from pure hoarding disorder. In hoarding disorder, the individual accumulates many items until they cannot use their house in a normal fashion, being unable, for example, to sit down, sleep, or bathe without moving objects. This accumulation is not due to obsessive fear but rather to extreme emotional attachment to the items.	There is some evidence that treatment with SSRI drugs or clomipramine may be helpful to some individuals. There is also some evidence that the addition of dopamine blocking drugs can also be useful.	People with hoarding disorder are often older and more likely to live alone than people with OCD.\n\nSome individuals give a history of an unhappy childhood with either a lack of love or a lack of money.\n\nPeople with hoarding disorder are often hugely embarrassed and ashamed of the way in which they live.

(cont.)

Table 8.1 (cont.)

Condition	What is it?	What are the main treatments?	Other points of interest
Hair pulling disorder	This is also known as trichotillomania. The individual feels a buildup of tension and gains relief by pulling out hair. This hair pulling can involve any hair on the body but most frequently involves hair on the head, eyebrows, and eyelashes.	Treatment known as 'habit reversal' can be useful for this condition. There are very few studies in this area. Overall, SSRI drugs or clomipramine are the most common treatment and may be helpful for some people. Dopamine blockers may also have a role. The drug N-acetylcysteine, which works on the glutamate system, has also been useful for some people with hair pulling disorder.	
Skin picking disorder	This is similar to hair pulling disorder because the individual usually describes a buildup of tension followed by relief when the self-harm has occurred.	In general, this has not been widely researched. Treatments are similar to those used for hair pulling disorder.	Sometimes the extent of this disorder and subsequent infection can be life-threatening.
OCD induced by drugs, illness, or another physical cause			Head injury and brain damage have been linked to this condition, as has the drug used in resistant schizophrenia, clozapine, in certain individuals.

Case Study 8.1

Siobhan is convinced her skin is a dreadful blotchy mess which disgusts and repulses people. In reality, there are very faint red marks on one cheek which are hardly noticeable. Because Siobhan worries so much about her skin, she always wears huge sunglasses and a scarf wrapped around her neck which also covers her cheeks. This apparel tends to cause people to look at her when she goes out on hot days. Siobhan, however, is convinced that people stare at her because they are repulsed by her skin.

People with BDD also often spend many hours gazing in the mirror. This has a tendency to increase their preoccupation and worry. If anyone stares in a mirror for a long time, they will eventually find something that they do not like about their appearance. Minor blemishes start to appear much more significant the more the person stares at them. People with BDD will also spend hours studying models and stars in magazines and on television.

BDD is a common condition, estimated to affect between 0.7 and 2.4 per cent of the population at any given time. The onset is usually in adolescence – a time when many people are preoccupied and unhappy with their appearance – but the condition mushrooms and continues from there. It is found in both men and woman, but it may be slightly more common in women. People with BDD often, but not always, have coexisting OCD. One of the problems with research on BDD is that people troubled by their appearance tend not to seek psychiatric or psychological help and instead visit dermatologists, facial surgeons, dentists, plastic surgeons, and other people whom they hope will correct their 'defect'. People with BDD are rarely happy with the outcome of such interventions, and many go on to request more and more procedures.

People with BDD often become very depressed, and there is a high rate of suicide attempts among them. First treatments of BDD focus on ERP models and encouraging the individual to face their fear without checking, mirror gazing, or other preventative measures. Typical checking and anxiety-reducing behaviours analogous to compulsive rituals include the following:

- Checking appearance in the mirror
- Camouflaging the perceived abnormality with makeup, posture, clothing, or hats
- Seeking reassurance from relatives and friends
- Skin picking to try to get rid of the flaw (consequently making the appearance much worse)
- Checking the imagined 'abnormality' by touching the affected area
- Seeking medical reassurance and cosmetic surgery by consulting dermatologists, cosmetic dentists, orthodontists, and cosmetic surgeons

Treatment of Body Dysmorphic Disorder

Treatment for BDD is very similar to that for OCD with some minor differences. Drug treatment with SSRIs or clomipramine has been shown to be useful in BDD. The effective doses are in the higher range of those recommended. ERP treatment for BDD involves facing the fear that people will be repulsed by their appearance by taking risks and not engaging in the anxiety-reducing behaviours listed previously. Although this is still the mainstay of treatment, cognitive interventions are also often used. This treatment is illustrated in the story of Ryan.

Case Study 8.2

Ryan, a 41-year-old man, was referred to the clinic by his general practitioner (GP), who was reluctant to refer Ryan for more surgery without a psychiatric opinion. Since his teens, Ryan has been convinced that his nose is too big. At age 35, he underwent a surgical operation to reduce the size of his nose (rhinoplasty). Initially, he felt better and gained more confidence, but then he began to worry that his nose was still rather large. He returned to the surgeon, who told Ryan that he could not recommend further operations. Ryan then went to see several doctors, all of whom told him there was nothing wrong with his nose. Due to this, Ryan became convinced that if he could afford to visit a cosmetic surgeon privately, he could obtain the 'perfect' nose. However, he had asked the GP to send him for one final opinion before he used his life's savings to have surgery. The GP refused to refer him unless Ryan agreed to a psychiatric assessment.

When he arrived for the appointment, Ryan was very unenthusiastic and did not want to engage with the therapist at all. He kept saying, 'If I just have the surgery I'll be OK'. The therapist suggested to him that he was unlikely to get further surgery and there was no evidence that the last surgery had helped. Cosmetic surgery is an imprecise science. One person's idea of a 'perfect' nose may differ greatly from another person's idea. Anyone seeking a 'perfect' nose is likely to be disappointed. Ryan believed this was wrong and that he definitely needed surgery (Figure 8.1). The therapist suggested two possible explanations for the way he was feeling:

- He had an extremely large nose which was ugly as he believed and was the cause of comment for everyone who saw him. The only way to rectify this situation would be for Ryan to have surgery.
- It was the way Ryan felt about his nose which caused the problem, and this fed into a vicious cycle.

Ryan listened to the therapist's theory but said he still believed that the first explanation was correct and that only surgery would correct it. He did, however, agree to have five sessions of CBT 'if only to convince my doctor that I really do need surgery'. The therapist agreed to this. Ryan appeared depressed and

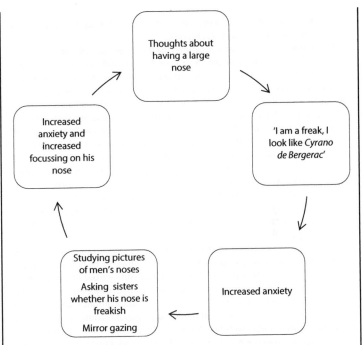

Figure 8.1 Cognitive behavioural model for Ryan's concerns regarding his nose

miserable, and the therapist was concerned about his low mood. Ryan admitted his mood had been low recently, but he believed this was purely due to the fact that he had not received surgery. Although he admitted to suicidal thoughts, he denied any plans but felt he might commit suicide if he did not ultimately get the surgery he believed he needed. The therapist suggested that his symptoms of depression may be helped by treatment with an SSRI, but Ryan was adamant that he did not need this. Ryan was asked to make a list of other men with large noses and bring it to the next session.

The following week, Ryan arrived with a list of people with large noses, including the French film actor Gerard Depardieu and other successful politicians and actors. The therapist asked Ryan what he noticed about these men. He replied, 'I know what you are going to say, yes, they all have big noses and yes, they have all had successful careers and success with women but that is different to me as my nose is much worse!' The therapist asked Ryan to bring some photographs of men he believed were attractive to the next session. For the remainder of this session, Ryan agreed to walk along the High Street with the therapist to observe how many people stared at Ryan's nose. The result of this was that contrary to Ryan's prediction, no one stared at his nose.

The next week, the therapist measured the length and breadth of Ryan's nose and also the length and breadth of his face. Ryan agreed that the nose should be in proportion with the face. From these figures was calculated the width and length ratio for his nose. Similar measurements were taken from the photographs which Ryan had brought. It was soon discovered that Ryan's nose was average in both length and width. Ryan dismissed this by saying that 'mine still looks much larger'. For homework this week, the therapist asked Ryan not to look in the mirror for more than five minutes three times a day and only to check his hair. In addition, he was asked to not telephone his sister for reassurance about his nose. Ryan did not believe that either of these requests was reasonable. A compromise was therefore reached whereby he would seek reassurance and mirror gaze as much as he liked on one day and record his anxiety throughout the day. On the second day, he was to carry out the programme as suggested by the therapist and record his anxiety. For the rest of the week, he could do whichever he believed was the most useful.

When Ryan returned the next week, his records showed that he felt better when he did not mirror gaze or seek reassurance. However, he had gone back to the mirror gazing and telephoning his sister for reassurance because he believed that by following the programme he was 'just trying to forget my problem'. The therapist proposed that Ryan walk around the hospital grounds and conduct a survey of people asking them what they thought about his nose. Ryan was fairly shy about this to begin with but did agree. Most people were complimentary about his nose, which was described as 'chiselled' and 'a fine Roman nose', and others were neither complimentary nor critical and said 'just looks normal'. After completing the survey, the therapist asked Ryan what he concluded from this exercise and he said, 'It does seem that the problem is more the thoughts about my nose rather than my nose'. From this point onwards, Ryan worked well in therapy, but he still did not wish to continue beyond five sessions. He agreed to reduce the time he spent in front of the mirror and to stop asking his sister for reassurance about his nose. He has decided to put his request to see a cosmetic surgeon 'on hold' for a while but says that although he is willing to try to 'live with my nose' for the next few months, he will seek surgery if his preoccupation with his nose increased again.

Ryan's story illustrates the use of ERP therapy for his BDD (i.e., going out in public and checking if people really stared at his nose and also asking people about his nose). This was also backed up with some cognitive work which involved testing his beliefs. So far, Ryan has resisted taking SSRI medication. However, these may help him feel better and to be able to face the challenge of treatment more readily.

Hoarding Disorder

Hoarding, or the accumulation of excessive numbers of items, is not a diagnosis by itself. Many people collect large numbers of items such as books, stamps, or ornaments. The difference between these collections and a 'hoard' is that generally a collection is organised in some way. Also, the collection does not normally threaten the individual's ability to function in the home or become a hazard.

Hoarding can be a result of many conditions. Physical illness and disability can mean that the person is unable to sort out their belongings. People with a learning disability or dementia may not be able to logically organise the items which come into their home. People who abuse substances such as alcohol or other drugs may have lost the ability to structure and control their lives. As previously discussed, hoarding may also be a feature of OCD.

Hoarding disorder refers to people who do not have any other complicating diagnosis or reason for accumulating their hoarded items. In these cases, people are frequently living in dangerous situations with risk of fire from hoarded items or even structural collapse of the property. Frequently, individuals are not referred to medical or psychiatric professions and are instead dealt with via the courts. Many are made homeless as a result of eviction due to their problems. These individuals can be very difficult to treat, and treatment can take a very long time. Unlike with OCD, drugs such as SSRIs and/or dopamine blockers may not have major beneficial effects. One of the most striking characteristics of patients with hoarding is their absolute belief that their hoards are 'valuable'. For example, an elderly woman who lived in a house which was falling down due to structural damage secondary to hoarded newspapers and letters suggested that for anyone to start throwing any of these items away was tantamount to 'committing grievous bodily harm to me'. Sufferers of pure hoarding disorder are more likely to be older than OCD sufferers (although they often give a history of the problem starting in childhood or adolescence) and to live alone, and many have a past history of childhood deprivation (either extreme poverty or emotional deprivation).

Treatment of Hoarding Disorder

It is not entirely clear whether or not SSRIs and drugs such as dopamine blockers are useful in hoarding disorder. Some studies claim that they do help, whereas others suggest they have little or no effect. One of the difficulties is that before 2013 and the publication of DSM-5, hoarding disorder was usually diagnosed as OCD. This means that many studies of people with hoarding also include people with OCD and hoarding symptoms. It is known that SSRIs and dopamine blockers can help people with OCD, but their effect on people with pure hoarding disorder is less clear.

Psychological treatment of hoarding is also based on an exposure type of model. People with hoarding disorder are often embarrassed and humiliated by their homes and the mess in which they live. They need to establish trust with their therapist and understand that this is not 'their fault' and that they are not 'lazy' or 'slovenly' but, rather, suffer from a psychological problem. Second, there needs to be an agreement that no more hoarded items must enter the house. It is pointless to start discarding items if more are being brought in. This is similar to trying to bail the water out of a sinking boat without mending the hole. Once trust has been established between patient and therapist and no further items are accumulated, it is time for the person to start discarding hoarded objects. Rules for determining whether objects should be discarded, recycled, or saved must be developed and agreed to by the patient. When making decisions about objects, the person with hoarding disorder should be encouraged to hold each object only once and not change their the decision once it is made. It appears that prolonged handling of an object leads to greater attachment of the individual to that object. Once an object is discarded, the hoarder is less distressed if they do not see the discarded item again.

Case Study 8.3

Albert is a 65-year-old unmarried man who lives alone in a housing association flat. He previously worked as a builder but retired five years ago. Referral was made to local psychiatric services via the housing association. Although the association was keen to help Albert, his excessive hoarding was putting other residents at risk of harm because objects had spilled out of his flat into communal areas, causing a risk that someone might fall. There was concern that the weight of his hoarded items would soon put the building structure at risk, and there was fear of fire due to the excessive papers, including in kitchen areas.

For the first meeting, Albert was insistent that he should meet the therapist at the hospital. He gave a history of a deprived and difficult childhood during which he had to move several times with his unmarried mother, who had had a series of relationships with different men. When he became an adult, he was determined to work to be able to afford 'nice' things in his home. Initially, he had managed to keep a tidy and functional home. He was married from the age of 25 to 50 years, but unfortunately his wife died of breast cancer 15 years ago. They had not had any children. Albert was distraught after his wife died, and he had never wished to form another relationship. Initially, he worked harder, but since taking retirement five years ago, he had found himself very lonely and isolated. His hoarding problem started soon after his wife died. He would visit various house clearance shops in his area and buy a variety of objects, mostly the type of objects or furniture which he remembered from his youth. In addition, he would buy multiple books in charity shops, although he rarely found the time to read them. In the first meeting, it was immediately apparent that Albert was very embarrassed by his problem. He described himself as 'lazy' and 'greedy' for having this problem. When it was suggested that the therapist might visit his home, Albert was adamant that this could not happen.

The first stage of therapy involved the therapist gaining Albert's trust. In addition, it was important to ensure that no more items were being brought into the house. The therapist discussed with Albert the feelings he had when he found a 'nice' item or a book. Albert described his excitement and pleasure at finding the item and said it gave him a 'buzz'; however, when he returned home, he felt humiliated and despondent that his flat was so overcrowded. It was clear that Albert lived a very sad and restricted life and that buying items was his chief pleasure, even though this led to deeper despair. It was important to establish a ban on new items coming into the house but also to try to ensure that Albert had some pleasurable activities to replace the excitement that resulted from his shopping. First, a discussion was held about Albert's interests. He admitted that he was very interested in reading and books. It was agreed that Albert would not visit any of his usual shops during the next week. When he went out to buy groceries, he would only take sufficient money (and no bank cards) to do this and not to buy anything else. In addition, he would go to the local library and find out about book reading clubs as well as sign up as a member so that he could borrow books.

For several weeks, Albert was resistant to the therapist visiting his home because he felt deeply ashamed about the state of his house. He was encouraged to take photographs of each room but was reluctant to do this. To start therapy, he was asked to bring a bag of items so that a decision could be made about them. Albert agreed that approximately 75 per cent of the items needed to be removed from his flat but was extremely anxious about doing so. At the next appointment, he arrived with a bag of books. Together with the therapist, he agreed that there were three categories of items:

1. Items for recycling for paper (rubbish): These were books with pages missing or which were badly torn or mouldy.

2. Items for disposal at charity shops/library: These were books in reasonably good condition but which he had read.

3. Items to keep: These were books of particular significance or value, such as first editions and family books inherited from his grandfather.

To this end, three large bags were made available for each of the three categories. Albert was then asked to take out a book and decide quickly which category it belonged in. It was important that he did not handle the item for too long because this tends to increase the attachment to an object. Also, it was negotiated that once a decision about disposal had been made, it was final. The session took two hours, and Albert found it extremely distressing and very difficult to discard items. During the session, he wept at times when discarding books and said he felt as if he was losing close friends. He was reminded of his goal of having a tidy, liveable flat with sufficient good-quality items for a comfortable life. Albert agreed to persevere, and at the end of the session, the therapist and Albert disposed of the bags in the recycling bin and at a local charity shop, leaving him with 2 books out of 30 which he wanted to take home. He was then given the task of continuing this process on his own until the next session.

After four weeks, Albert had progressed well and had discarded several large bags full of books. He had had one setback when he had gone back to the charity shop and said he had changed his mind, but the books had already been sent to a central sorting office. The therapist praised Albert for his progress but said the next session would have to be in Albert's home.

At the first home-based session, six weeks after starting therapy, the therapist first had to gauge the risk to both Albert and herself. There have been reported incidents in which people have been killed or seriously injured due to items falling on the hoarder. Clearly, the risk of this occurring increases once items are starting to be moved. Other risks to the therapist include health risks from extreme dirt and squalor, risk of building collapse, or risk of being trapped and fire. Any person entering such an environment, whether a professional called to help with the problem or a friend or relative, must ensure their own health and safety, as well as that of the person who hoards. In the rarest and most serious cases, if there is a serious risk to health and safety, then it may be necessary to consider legal enforcement and clearing of the property; there must also be consideration of whether the Mental Health Act is appropriate. It is often necessary for the therapist to wear protective overalls and a mask because of dust and dirt.

In this case, although the hoarding was severe, there was no immediate danger, and Albert agreed not to use the cooker until the kitchen was cleared of fire hazards. First, the therapist gained Albert's permission to take photographs of the different rooms. The house was almost completely full, with piles of items covering approximately 80 per cent of all available floor space. In the kitchen, books were piled up on every work surface, and there was a risk of fire from books being piled next to the cooker. His bed was also covered, with just a small space on the edge for him to sleep. The bath was piled high with books; Albert had been unable to take a bath for several years. The living room had a small space with one chair and a television, but there was only a narrow passageway through stacks of items to reach these.

Work started on clearing the kitchen, using the same categories for items as before. Again, this was very difficult for Albert, but he began to feel encouraged as he saw the space around his cooker getting cleared and the work surfaces which he had not seen for several years started to appear.

Treating a hoarder such as Albert is a lengthy and painstaking process. Most cases will take many months, and it is not unusual for them to take a year. In these cases, it is unrealistic to expect a therapist to attend weekly for many hours to allow clearing to take place. Consideration should be given to enlisting a 'co-therapist' who may be a mental health worker, a 'befriender' from the local mental health services, or a family member or friend. The co-therapist needs to have the trust of the patient and also needs to understand the rules for the treatment:

- There is a ban on new items coming into the house.
- Each item is allocated to the 'Discard', 'Charity Shop', or 'Keep' bag.
- Each item is held for a few seconds (no more than two minutes) for a decision to be made.

- Items must only be handled once (i.e., no going back on decisions)
- Once sorted, the items are disposed of immediately following the session.

In Albert's case, he began working with a befriender from his local community mental health team who agreed to visit once a week and help him discard his items. If they managed to clear as much as they had hoped, they would then go out for a coffee after having dropped items off at the charity shop. The therapist contacted them every few weeks to ensure progress and to troubleshoot any difficulties. Albert finished clearing his home 15 months after the first appointment. The local social services arranged for his flat to be 'deep-cleaned'.

Albert is now delighted with his new living situation but needs to think about relapse prevention. The therapist and Albert have developed the following plan to prevent the same situation from recurring:

- I will continue to borrow books from the library and attend the reading groups there.
- I have purchased an electronic book reader and so will no longer buy paper books.
- I will restrict my cash and bank cards when going out and only buy what I have previously decided and take money for those items only.
- If I do purchase a new item or new piece of furniture, *something of equivalent size has to be discarded.*

Albert's story demonstrates that people with hoarding disorder can often be helped but that they need to accept that they have a problem and wish to work to overcome the problem. Treatment is often lengthy, but the long-term results can be truly life-changing.

Tourette's Syndrome and Tics

Tourette's syndrome is a neurological condition which starts in childhood and continues into adulthood. Many people with Tourette's syndrome spontaneously get better after approximately ten years of the condition, but approximately one-third of people have a long-term condition which does tend to get better as they age. The condition is characterised by a combination of involuntary noises and also movements known as tics. It can often be associated with attention-deficit/hyperactivity disorder, in which the individual is restless and has difficulties concentrating, and also with OCD. The tics which are seen may be vocal (sounds; e.g., coughing, grunting, or shouting out words) or physical (movements; e.g., sudden movements of the arms or legs, jerking of the head, or jumping up and down). In addition, tics may be simple (e.g., making a small jerky movement or uttering a single sound) or complex (e.g., making a series of movements or speaking a phrase).

It is thought that Tourette's syndrome is due to abnormalities arising in the basal ganglia area of the brain. This is the same areas that is thought to be involved in OCD.

It can often be difficult to distinguish between a complex tic and a compulsive ritual. In a complex tic, the urge to perform the tic comes on and becomes increasingly stronger until the tic is performed. Compulsive rituals are performed in response to a specific and unpleasant obsessive thought.

Tics and Tourette's syndrome often result in children being teased and bullied; therefore, rapid treatment is a necessity to help these children socially develop.

Treatment of Tourette's Syndrome and Tics

Some of the drugs used to treat Tourette's syndrome and tics are listed in Table 8.2.

Table 8.2 Examples of the variety of drug treatments used for Tourette's syndrome

Type of drug	Examples (not comprehensive)	Trade names	Notes
Dopamine blockers			
	Haloperidol	Haldol, Dozic, Serenace	Used for many years but is one of the traditional, older dopamine blockers. Can have side effects including sedation and drowsiness, prolonged muscle contraction, stiffness, and shakiness.
	Pimozide	Orap	Another traditional dopamine blocker with similar but fewer side effects compared to haloperidol.
	Aripiprazole	Abilify	An atypical (newer) dopamine blocker and is often the drug used first for Tourette's syndrome because it is generally well tolerated. Side effects are usually mild to moderate and often pass as the drug is continues. Common side effects include restlessness, insomnia or drowsiness, fatigue, nausea, and headaches.
	Rispiridone	Risperdal	Another atypical dopamine blocking drug. This has been investigated extensively, with many studies reporting positive effects. Side effects include fatigue and somnolence, emotional disturbance, nausea, vomiting, sleep problems, and weight gain.

Table 8.2 (cont.)

Type of drug	Examples (not comprehensive)	Trade names	Notes
Alpha-2 adrenergic agonists			
	Clonidine	Catapres, Dixarit	This has been prescribed for many years for the treatment of tics in childhood. Possible side effects include drowsiness, sedation, headaches, depression, dizziness, and a drop in blood pressure. People need to have their blood pressure checked before taking and whilst on clonidine.
Muscle relaxants			
	Baclofen	Lyflex	Main side effects are drowsiness and dizziness. Adults need to avoid alcohol, and if they are affected with drowsiness and dizziness, they should not drive nor operate machinery.
	Clonazepam		Main side effects are drowsiness and dizziness. Adults need to avoid alcohol, and if they are affected with drowsiness and dizziness, they should not drive nor operate machinery.

Psychological treatment used for tic disorder and Tourette's syndrome usually involves a treatment known as habit reversal, although people with OCD will also need treatment using ERP. Habit reversal treatment has four components:

1. Awareness training
2. Competing response training
3. Habit control motivation
4. Generalisation training

Case Study 8.4

Sarah, an attractive and lively 24-year-old games mistress, was referred to the clinic with a 14-year history of unsightly and embarrassing facial tics. The onset occurred at puberty, but it was not related by Sarah to any particular life event. Throughout the years, she had received treatment with a variety of medications, including haloperidol and muscle relaxant drugs, with partial effect.

The tic can occur at any time but is more frequent if she is anxious or bored. Close observation of the movements revealed that it commences with Sarah screwing up both eyes, followed by crinkling her nose and then making a sharp downward movement of her chin opening her mouth.

Sarah was first asked to record the frequency of her tics over a few days. This *awareness training* is useful because many people with habit disorders are oblivious to some of the times when they perform the undesirable behaviour. Obviously, Sarah has a busy life and so the records were made as simple as possible for her to keep. She was asked to obtain a small notebook and to divide each page into columns, each representing a one-hour period. Every time she performed the tic, she was to place a mark in the appropriate column. Also, she was to record her activity at each hourly interval – for example, 'lunch with colleagues' and 'netball lesson with Lower Sixth Form'.

This diary was also useful as a baseline measure of Sarah's problem, and it was maintained throughout treatment to monitor her progress. The baseline measures showed that Sarah performed the tic an average of 300 times a day or approximately 0.5 tics per minute.

At the second session, the principle of competing response practice was explained to Sarah. The therapist said,

> One of the problems with a long-standing habit is that you have built up and strengthened the muscles of your face which are involved in the tic at the expense of the opposing muscles. What I will be asking you to do is to perform some exercises to strengthen these opposing muscles. The start of every tic begins with you screwing up both your eyes. As soon as you feel that you are going to tic, I want you to raise your eyebrows, wrinkling your forehead. You may find this easier to do if you place your thumb and index finger of one hand under each of your eyebrows. I then want you to hold this position to the count of 20 or until the urge to tic passes, whichever is the longer time. At the same time as doing this, I would like you to clench you teeth together very tightly and likewise to maintain this position.

Following this description, the therapist asked Sarah to practice the competing response in the session. The therapist then asked Sarah to list all the negative effects of having a tic and the advantages of being tic-free. She was asked to write this list down and to read it whenever she felt bored or disheartened by the treatment (*habit control motivation*).

Finally, ways in which Sarah could incorporate the competing response movements into her everyday life without looking conspicuous were discussed. Sarah suggested that if she were outside, she could place her hand under her eyebrows as if shielding her eyes from the sun. If she were inside and sitting at a desk or table, she could use her hand under her eyebrows to 'support' her head (*generalisation training*).

When Sarah was seen a week later for her third session, the frequency of tics had already reduced to less than 10 per cent of the baseline level. Difficulties were discussed with her during this session and also during the following two sessions.

Six weeks after starting the treatment, Sarah was discharged from the clinic. Her tics are now occurring less than five times a day, and she believes they are controllable.

Hair Pulling Disorder (Trichotillomania)

Hair pulling disorder is sometimes known as 'trichotillomania'. People with this condition pull out the hair on their heads or sometimes eyebrows and eyelashes. Rarely does this disorder involve body hair. People with this condition often describe a pleasurable feeling of satisfaction if they have had a 'good' hair pulling session even though they are distressed about the effect of hair loss on their appearance. Some people describe being distracted and not noticing when they are hair pulling. This condition is more common in teenagers, and it tends to affect more girls than boys. Stress is a frequent precursor to the hair pulling.

Many people who have hair pulling disorder do not seek psychological help but instead may be referred to dermatologists or trichologists. Due to a feeling of shame, many do not admit to the hair pulling and thus often do not receive the help they need.

A serious and even life-threatening consequence for some people who hair pull and then swallow the hair is that the hair cannot be easily digested and can form large balls in the gut which can lead to blockages requiring emergency surgery.

Treatment of Hair Pulling Disorder

Drug treatment for hair pulling disorder is based mostly on small trials involving small numbers of people, so it is difficult to determine the effectiveness of the treatment . The four main types of drug treatment are SSRI drugs, drugs which act as dopamine blockers, drugs which act on the 'addiction' pathways of the brain, and drugs which act on the glutamate system (see Chapter 4). None of these drug treatments, however, has been fully evaluated; thus, it is difficult to recommend them. SSRIs are likely to be useful if the person also has symptoms of OCD. Whereas some early studies suggested that SSRIs helped reduce hair pulling behaviours, more recent studies have raised doubt as to whether this is really the case. Studies on dopamine blockers (see Chapter 4) also have shown mixed results, with some studies finding them useful and others not. Hair pulling can be viewed as an 'impulse control disorder' because the act of hair pulling is usually described as pleasurable, even though the consequences are upsetting to the individual. Thus, it has been thought that it may have some similarities, in terms of brain chemistry, with a variety of conditions, including alcohol and drug abuse, addictive gambling, smoking, and kleptomania (addictive stealing). Naltrexone is a drug which is thought to block some of the pleasure centres in the brain which are activated by problematic addictive behaviours. There is some indication that naltrexone may be useful for some people with hair pulling disorder. In terms of drugs which act on the glutamate system, *N*-acetylcysteine has been reported to be useful for some people with hair pulling disorder. This drug was originally used for paracetamol overdose and to loosen mucous in people with cystic fibrosis or chronic lung disease. It was found to be active on the glutamate system and has been tried for several conditions related to OCD but is most notably used for hair pulling disorder. Despite a number of trials suggesting that it may be useful, these trials involved small numbers of patients and so it is not possible to fully endorse its use. It is generally well tolerated with few side effects and therefore may be worth trying.

Treatment to deal with the underlying stress and/or depression may be needed, as might family therapy to deal with family tensions. For many people, however, the hair pulling itself is the main cause of stress and family tension. Psychological treatment is mainly habit reversal training. This treatment was described in the section on tic disorder and Tourette's syndrome. In hair pulling, it consists of the same four components:

1. Awareness training: Whereas some people with hair pulling disorder do set out to have a 'hair pulling session' to reduce stress and tension, many are unaware of their habit most of the time. Part of the treatment is to closely monitor the behaviour and also to note where they are and what they are doing when it occurs. Although many people will say there are no obvious precipitants to the behaviour, carefully recording in this way can show patterns and stressors of which they were previously unaware. Collecting and keeping all the pulled hair is also useful and, in itself, has often shocked individuals into trying to radically change their behaviour.

2. Competing response training: Forming a fist and keeping it tightly closed or other similar activities which are incompatible with hair pulling may be used. Wearing a hat, or even a wig, can also form a barrier to prevent hair pulling from occurring.

3. Habit control motivation: Like any treatment, habit reversal requires motivation and commitment. Recording all the negative factors about the problem can be very useful. This list should be written on a piece of paper or recorded on a cell phone so it can be read or listened to when there is an urge to pull hair.

4. Generalisation training: Incorporating the response into everyday life can be helpful. For example, a woman who worked as a waitress decided that instead of forming a fist, she would sharply grip the tray she was carrying when she had an urge to pull her hair.

Skin Picking

Skin picking disorder is another condition described in the DSM-5 as one of the obsessive–compulsive and related disorders. Many people with the condition do not seek help from psychiatrists or psychologists, preferring to attend dermatology clinics. Diagnosis can sometimes be difficult because many people do not like to admit the condition is self-inflicted. Skin picking is a symptom and may be part of another condition, such as the following:

- Body dysmorphic disorder, where skin picking is an attempt to reduce the perceived blemish on the skin (but inevitably makes it worse)
- OCD, where the person picks at the skin to remove 'dirt'

- Acne, where people skin pick and squeeze spots in an attempt to make them reduce (again making the situation worse)
- Either during or following withdrawal of certain illegal or prescribed stimulant drugs
- As an accompaniment to a delusional belief that the individual is infested by parasites which they then try to remove

These conditions all require different treatment, but skin picking can be a disorder in its own right. The severity of the disorder can range from minimal to life-threatening when an individual renders themselves prone to infections.

Treatment of Skin Picking

The studies of drug treatment of skin picking disorder have all been small, and it is difficult to give definitive advice. Studies on SSRIs for skin picking have shown mixed results, with some showing improvement and some no response. Drugs acting on the glutamatergic system have been tried, and individual case reports have suggested that N-acetylcysteine may be beneficial.

Psychological treatment for skin picking is based on habit reversal techniques (identical to those used for hair pulling and tic disorders). Again, studies are small but seem to show that this kind of approach is beneficial. Some people have combined habit reversal techniques with some cognitive therapy to good effect.

Health Anxiety

Health anxiety is not classified as an obsessive–compulsive and related disorder but it does display many of the same characteristics as OCD.

Health anxiety refers to individuals who are constantly worrying about their health. Some people focus on one particular condition, such as cancer or heart disease. Others interpret every small change in their body as being due to a dreadful disease. These worrying thoughts come into the person's mind, and they may then start checking behaviours such as checking for lumps or feeling their pulse. They may also ask for reassurance from their loved ones, or may repeatedly visit the GP or hospital for reassurance. These checks and reassurance are identical to the situation seen with OCD, and so they reduce the anxiety slightly, but the effect is short-lived and the person then seeks more reassurance. Some people with health anxiety therefore become 'blacklisted' at their GP's office, the local accident and emergency department, or walk-in centres. Rather like the boy who always cried wolf, they establish the worst-case scenario for themselves so that they find it difficult to obtain help when they really need it.

All of us experience a range of physical symptoms every day, most of which are not indicative of serious disease. Once someone focuses on a symptom, however, this will generally make it worse. To test this out, try sitting quietly and concentrate on your right big toe and imagine it is painful. Eventually, most people will experience pain in their toe if they concentrate in this way. In the same way, overconcentrating on any bodily symptom will tend to increase this symptom. If individuals with health anxiety can be taught to view their symptoms in another way, they will often improve.

Treatment of Health Anxiety

Although only a small number of studies of drug treatment in health anxiety have been conducted, it appears that SSRIs are useful. Unfortunately, however, many people with health anxiety are very sensitive to any bodily symptoms, including side effects of drugs. It is thus best to start on lower doses and increase gradually.

Psychological treatment involves ERP combined with some cognitive interventions.

Case Study 8.5

Ash is a 25-year-old man who was referred for assessment by the gastroenterology team. He was extremely reluctant to see a psychiatrist but was eventually persuaded by being told that many patients benefit from seeing the psychiatrist irrespective of their diagnosis, as any emotion can have an effect on the bowel.

The history showed that Ash is the only child of quite elderly parents, who had undergone many attempts at in vitro fertilisation to conceive him. Consequently, he had been quite 'molly-coddled' as a young child and was always described as 'sickly', requiring considerable time away from school, although no serious pathology had ever been found.

At age 18 years, Ash moved away from home to attend university. He developed some abdominal pains and went to the student health centre. He was told that this was most likely due to his poor diet since leaving home. Ash, however, was not happy with this answer and started searching the Internet. He convinced himself that he suffered from a form of ulcerative colitis and that he would die from the complications of carcinoma unless this was dealt with. After several visits to the health centre, he was sent to the hospital to see a gastroenterologist. The consultant at the clinic performed a sigmoidoscopy on Ash and reassured him there was nothing wrong. Initially, Ash was relieved, but during the next few days he was plagued by thoughts such as the following:

- 'Doctors can get things wrong. What if he missed the pathological area?'
- 'I only had sigmoidoscopy and that can only examine the lower bowel. Maybe the upper bowl is affected.'
- 'Maybe he's only telling me there's nothing wrong because he thinks I'm really ill and the prognosis is hopeless.'

These thoughts caused Ash to ask for an urgent return visit to the clinic and eventually was given a colonoscopy. Each new test reduced his anxiety for a while, but then the catastrophic thoughts would creep back in. Eventually, the local clinic refused to see him. By this time, Ash was so crippled by his anxieties that he was no longer attending to his studies. He returned home, where his parents were very concerned about his weight loss. Ash had started to restrict his diet to that advised for people with ulcerative colitis and so was avoiding most sources of insoluble fibre (e.g., bran, whole foods, and sweet corn) and also any dairy produce, including milk, cheese, and cream. As well as trying to avoid physical activity in case it upset his bowel, Ash took a variety of tablets from health food shops, consisting of a range of vitamin and mineral supplements and also Chinese medicines supposed to act on the bowel. During the next few years, Ash had more investigations and saw a multiplicity of National Health Service and private gastroenterologists. Every time he was discharged from a clinic, his anxiety would skyrocket and he would seek out another physician and surgeon. At the time of referral to the psychiatric clinic, Ash had a body mass index of only 16, and he spent most of his days lying in bed. He was pale and unwell, and he spent his time searching the Internet for a cure for his 'ulcerative colitis'. His parents were extremely anxious and really did believe Ash had a serious medical condition. His mother said, 'Look at the state of him, he's undernourished and can barely get out of bed. There must be something seriously wrong with him that the doctors haven't found'. The family had spent more than £10,000, which they could barely afford, to try to get a diagnosis for Ash.

The case history of Ash demonstrates how medical practitioners unwittingly exacerbate the symptoms of health anxiety. Most patients will attend their GP office or hospital clinic and accept the outcome of relevant tests. However, medicine is not an exact science, and there are hardly any situations in which a doctor can honestly say he or she is 100 per cent certain. If a patient returns and becomes insistent, then the doctor, mindful of the potential for medicolegal allegations and negligence claims if a diagnosis is overlooked, will often concede to the patient's demands and order further tests. As can be seen from Ash's history, this can form a vicious cycle with a downward spiral of the patient.

In treating patients with health anxiety, the psychiatrist must first establish with the patient that there will be no more medical tests or seeking of reassurance for the duration of psychological treatment. This is easier said than done. Patients with health anxiety really believe they have a serious physical illness which may threaten their lives, and so it will seem as if the therapist is asking them to take a major risk. One way of approaching this is to present two scenarios to the patient. This can be demonstrated in the story of the treatment of Ash.

Case Study 8.5 (cont.)

At first, Ash was very unwilling to agree to stop consulting doctors about his bowels. He believed this would be 'dangerous' and that his symptoms might progress and worsen, but the therapist said,

I understand your concern about you bowls but if we look at this, you have been seeking a diagnosis for over 7 years now. I am asking you to agree to no further investigations for the next 4 months whilst we start to look at alternative answers. I am going to propose to you that there are two possible explanations for your situation.

Firstly, your current belief is that you have a serious bowel condition such as ulcerative colitis and that this will result in a life-threatening situation. All the doctors and specialists who have seen you have managed to miss this diagnosis, but if you keep on seeing more specialists and having more tests, you will eventually obtain a diagnosis of inflammatory bowel disease.

My theory is that you do indeed suffer from a variety of bowel symptoms. These symptoms may well have been precipitated originally by a poor diet when you left home. However, once you became anxious that you had a serious bowel disease, your anxiety increased. Chronic and high anxiety can cause various symptoms which you describe, such as colicky pain, intermittent diarrhoea and constipation, and a feeling of nausea. Every time you go and see a specialist, you feel better for a day or two, and then start to worry they may have overlooked the diagnosis and your anxiety and symptoms get worse. In addition, your restricted diet has made you severely underweight. This diet may well be contributing to your bowel symptoms and also being malnourished means you will have low energy, lack of drive, and feeling of malaise. This in turn leads you to spend increasing time in bed. Remaining in bed makes you weaker and also has a deleterious effect on your physical symptoms.

Ash did not agree with the therapist's theory but, persuaded by his parents, agreed to give it a try, and he also agreed that he would not consult any bowel specialist for the next six weeks. The therapist gave him a chart to take away (Figure 8.2). He also agreed to stop the Chinese medicine but decided to remain on the vitamin supplements.

In therapy, the first task was to try to modify some of Ash's beliefs about his symptoms. He was asked to search the Internet to identify some of the symptoms caused by anxiety and determine if any of these matched the ones he had. Over the next few sessions, the emphasis was placed on examining Ash's symptoms and thoughts and, by working jointly with Ash, trying to discover if there were any alternative explanations other than serious bowel disease for his symptoms. At the end of several sessions, Ash conceded that his belief that his symptoms were caused by anxiety had increased from 0 to 40 per cent. He was asked if he would be willing to try expanding the repertoire of his diet. After a long discussion, Ash agreed to include dairy produce in his diet for a week to determine if this caused his symptoms to improve or deteriorate.

Ash managed to incorporate dairy produce without ill effect and was successfully challenging many of his thoughts concerning serious bowel disease. He was already spending less time in bed, but the therapist worked with him to consider

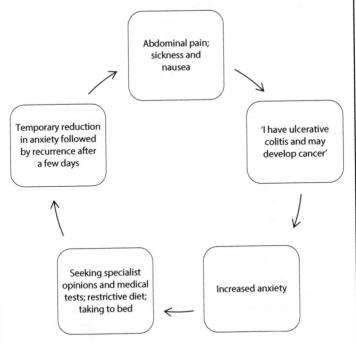

Figure 8.2 Ash's chart

introducing graded exercise to gradually increase his physical activity. He found that as he grew stronger and was eating a better diet, his symptoms were less prominent. After several weeks, he agreed to eat wholemeal and foods rich in fibre. Once a full and varied diet was established, he agreed to stop his vitamin and mineral supplements.

Ash started some more detailed work with the therapist examining some of his thoughts and the deeper beliefs that he held about his health and fitness. Many of these were successfully challenged, and he stopped viewing himself as weak and sickly and began to understand that he could be a strong and healthy man. Following on from this, Ash decided to try to take up judo. He enrolled in a local class, and to his surprise, he not only enjoyed the sport but also was reasonably good at it.

Currently, Ash looks like a strong, fit, healthy, and happy young man. He no longer restricts his diet, although he does try to maintain a healthy diet, which he believes helps him perform better in judo competitions.

The case of Ash demonstrates how people with health anxiety can be helped to overcome their problems. Not everyone is as willing to try to engage in therapy and to 'take the risk' that some of their symptoms may be related to anxiety and to some of the behaviours they are using to try to prevent ill health. People who engage with the effort to complete therapy can be dramatically improved and feel much better both physically and emotionally.

Key Points

- Body dysmorphic disorder (BDD) has many similarities to OCD, and frequently both OCD and BDD coexist.

- Treatment for BDD involves SSRIs as for OCD and also ERP. In addition, some cognitive techniques are often needed for BDD.

- Hoarding can be a symptom of several psychiatric and physical conditions.

- In hoarding disorder, an individual is unable to stop acquiring a huge number of possessions and is unable to dispose of the excess. This condition may be associated with a deprived upbringing (either materially or emotionally deprived).

- Hoarding disorder results in considerable shame and embarrassment, and those working with a person who has hoarding disorder need to gain the person's trust. Health and safety issues must always take precedence. The danger to the person with hoarding disorder, their neighbours, and the public, as well as the therapist involved in helping them, must be taken into account.

- Treatment for hoarding disorder may involve SSRIs and possibly dopamine blockers.

- The mainstay of treatment for hoarding disorder is CBT involving a ban on the acquisition of any new items and a programme of controlled discarding of excess items.

- Tourette's syndrome involves vocal and/or physical tics. This condition often coexists with OCD or attention-deficit/hyperactivity disorder.

- Drug treatment for Tourette's syndrome involves dopamine blocking drugs such as haloperidol or the newer aripiprazole. Alpha-2 adrenergic blockers or muscle relaxants may also be useful.

- Psychological treatment for both Tourette's syndrome and tic disorder involves habit reversal.

- Habit reversal consists of the following:
    - Awareness training
    - Competing response training

- · Habit control motivation
- · Generalisation training
- Hair pulling and skin picking disorders are more recently recognised conditions. For both disorders, only small-scale research examining their treatment has been performed. SSRIs have shown mixed results in studies. More novel agents such as *N*-acetylcysteine (a glutamate modulator) may be useful. Naltrexone may also prove useful. Psychological treatment for both disorders involves habit reversal.
- Health anxiety is very similar to OCD with anxious thoughts leading to compulsive rituals and reassurance seeking.
- Only very small studies of drug treatment for health anxiety have been performed. SSRIs are the drugs of choice. Sometimes it is wise to start at a low dose and build up because people with health anxiety can be very sensitive to any change in their body and to side effects.
- Psychological treatment of health anxiety involves ERP combined with some cognitive interventions.

References

1. American Psychiatric Association. (2013). *Diagnostic and Statistical Manual of Mental Disorders* (5th ed.). Arlington, VA: American Psychiatric Publishing.
2. World Health Organisation. (1993). *The ICD 10 Classification of Mental and Behavioural Disorders: Diagnostic Criteria for Research*. Geneva, Switzerland: Author.

What Can Family and Carers Do to Help a Person with OCD?

This chapter will examine what family members and carers can do to help someone with OCD. In the case of the parents of a person with OCD, the natural reaction is to try to prevent their offspring from experiencing extreme anxiety and distress. This reaction means they can often get caught up being asked to participate in OCD compulsions and rituals and also to obey many of the 'rules' which people with OCD may devise to avoid setting off OCD thoughts. Despite the fact that this compliance with the OCD rituals is done by the carers with the best of intentions, it serves to actually worsen the OCD symptoms over time. It can often be useful for carers to realise that they are the people without OCD, and thus they need to set the 'ground rules' of what they will or will not tolerate and do in their own home. However, in many cases, this is easier said than done. First, old habits die hard. Second, it can be extremely difficult to resist stepping in if a loved-one is highly distressed. This will be explored in this chapter as well as possible solutions.

Throughout this chapter, it is emphasised that the safety of any children, other family members, and the person with OCD is paramount. When an individual suffers from OCD, they can become very distressed and agitated when having extreme obsessive symptoms. A minority of these people may become violent at these times. Violence is never acceptable, and family, carers, and friends have a duty to themselves and also to the person with OCD to keep themselves safe at all times. This may require families to request help from the police in extreme cases. As stated at the beginning, children are the paramount consideration. They may be harmed not only by violent actions but also by being asked to engage in OCD activities and being required to have a restricted life rather than be outside playing with friends or inviting friends to their home. This can be a difficult area for the OCD sufferer and those around them, but it is vital that the welfare of any children is always considered first and foremost.

As demonstrated in previous chapters and through the case studies of OCD sufferers, OCD is a problem which has a huge impact on the whole family. Severe OCD can result in a delay of normal maturation, with a young person living at home dependent on their parents and siblings for decades. On the other hand, many people with severe OCD are unable to work and unable to form long-lasting relationships. Many live alone and lead isolated and restricted lives, which can also cause worry and concern to friends and relatives.

One of the main problems of living with a person with OCD is knowing how to deal with their obsessions and compulsions. Family members may be asked for constant reassurance, asked to carry out activities which the person with OCD finds difficult, and often asked to carry out compulsive rituals. These requests and demands can cause major problems in families. Family members do not wish to see a loved one disturbed and upset and will understandably try to do everything they can to reduce the distress. As previously discussed, the problem is that reassurance-seeking or the completion of compulsive rituals may temporarily reduce the discomfort and anxiety, but this effect is short-lived and very soon more requests and demands are made. Similarly, it can often seem easier for family members to take on tasks and chores to help the person with OCD, but this can also escalate. A question I am often asked by relatives of people with OCD is how they should work with the person with OCD to prevent themselves from being dragged into the 'OCD quagmire'.

It is very important that family members not blame themselves for trying to help their loved one. This is a normal and natural reaction, and any caring person would do whatever they could to try to prevent the distress caused by OCD. It can be heartbreaking to witness the emotional turmoil being experienced by a loved-one. It would not be helpful or prudent for someone who has been providing reassurance and help to suddenly stop doing so. Full and frank discussions need to be held both with the person who has OCD and with other family members. First, the other family members need to establish in their own minds what is 'reasonable'. This may take some time to work out. OCD can often creep up gradually, and suddenly people find themselves living very restrictive lives with their relative with OCD. What has become 'normal' is far from normal in fact. However, it can be difficult to realise this when living with someone with OCD, and so it is worthwhile taking time to think through what is and what is not acceptable. If available, it can be useful to discuss this with another person who is outside the family, such as a general practitioner or a counsellor, who can help establish some ideas for the family. If a family member has OCD and is under the care of mental health services, their relatives can ask for a 'carer's assessment', in which their own problems and needs are assessed and help such as counselling can be offered.

Some relatives may find the obsessive fears so difficult to understand or so exaggerated that they are tempted to ridicule or belittle the fears. It is extremely important, however, to recognise that these thoughts are profoundly disturbing to the individual with OCD and are therefore extremely serious in their mind. Although they may realise their thoughts are either irrational or exaggerated, the fear accompanying these thoughts is very real and they are unable to 'snap out of it'. Instead, family and friends need to listen and try to understand what their loved one is experiencing.

A discussion must be held with the person who has OCD and their family members to ensure everyone involved understands OCD and that reassurance and compulsive rituals only temporarily help the symptoms of OCD and serve to increase symptoms in the long term. It is essential that everyone is open and clear about this as otherwise if reassurance and help with compulsions are suddenly withdrawn, it can feel like punishment to the person with OCD. It must also be clear that the ultimate responsibility for overcoming OCD lies with the person who has it. Other family members need to care for themselves and their own health and well-being. Although they will be supportive to their relative, they cannot take responsibility for their relative's treatment. Of course, the situation is different with a child who has OCD, in which case the parent has to assume much more responsibility in helping the child overcome OCD (see Chapter 6).

Once the ground rules have been established within the family, it is then time to try to implement them. This is unlikely to be a smooth ride. First, old habits die hard, and it is very easy for all family members to slip back into old routines. Second, the person with OCD may temporarily become more distressed, and this can make it very difficult to resist. It is vital that there be no violence or threats from anyone. Violence and similar behaviours are fully discussed later in this chapter.

Case Study 9.1

Violet, a 30-year-old woman, lives with her parents, who are both in their Sixties, in a house in a small market town. She was a much wanted child who was born after her parents had been told that they were unlikely to ever have children. Consequently, she was always rather 'spoiled' and was used to getting her own way. At the age of 11, she developed a fear of dirt and germs. This led to excessive washing and cleaning behaviours. In order to prevent distress to her daughter, Violet's mother did everything Violet asked her to do. At the time she was first seen in the clinic, Violet ruled her entire house. Her father had taken early retirement to care for Violet, and her mother had not worked since Violet was born. Most of their time was spent indoors, and her mother had a list of daily cleaning which Violet expected her to perform. If Violet did not believe this cleaning was performed 'properly', then she would demand her mother repeat the entire process. Occasionally, Violet's demands resulted in her mother cleaning for eight hours a day. Feeling unable to wash and care for herself, Violet also insisted that her mother wash her. She would stand in the shower whilst her mother cleaned her with antibacterial shower gel. Again, if Violet believed this was not performed 'properly', she would demand that her mother repeat it until she felt 'right'. Going to the toilet would take Violet up to an hour to urinate and four hours to defaecate. She performed these activities alone, but she demanded absolute silence in the house when these occurred. The slightest noise would result in her repeating her compulsions again and taking even longer. Her father was only allowed to leave the house when Violet gave 'permission', and when he returned with shopping or other items, a strict 'decontamination' procedure of all items was demanded by Violet. The family rarely left the house but every year spend two weeks in a holiday camp in July, which had done for more than 20 years. Whilst away, there was little evidence of Violet's OCD, but it would return as soon as she came home.

Violet's story demonstrates the absolute control that a person with OCD can inflict on a household. Both parents were keen to 'do what was right' for their daughter, but in trying to avoid upsetting her, they had made the situation worse. The story also shows another interesting observation for some people with OCD: Their symptoms can sometimes 'disappear' in a new environment. Unfortunately, they will return the longer the person remains in this different environment. In other words, if Violet's family had remained in the holiday camp environment, her OCD would have gradually returned over the next weeks.

In this case, it is likely to be hopeless to work with just Violet. Her parents have adapted their whole lifestyle around her OCD. Indeed, in a case such as this in which the situation has developed over decades, it is often necessary to move those like Violet into a new environment away from her parents to work on her OCD treatment. Meanwhile, her parents would receive help to try to re-establish their own 'normal' life.

Case Study 9.1 (cont.)

A trial of inpatient treatment was offered to Violet. She was insistent that she would not move away from home. When her parents urged her to accept the treatment, pointing out that they were not going to be around forever to do everything for her, Violet responded saying, 'Well, I will then get myself a maid'. Because Violet refused to engage in any therapy, the therapist started to work with the family and to encourage the parents to establish 'ground rules' of what they would and would not tolerate. First, her mother said she was uncomfortable washing a 30-year-old woman. This was explained to Violet. The first time her mother refused to wash her and Violet was told to just stand in the shower if she could not wash herself, Violet screamed and cried for two hours. Her parents did not respond, and she eventually left the shower unassisted. This situation was extremely difficult for Violet's mother, Doris, who found herself unable to resist Violet's demands because she did not wish to see her daughter in a distressed state. Violet's care coordinator therefore arranged for her mother to have a carer's assessment to identify the support she needed. For the carer's assessment, Doris was offered an appointment at the community health team. She was seen by a member of the team, and it was agreed that whilst she was going through such a stressful period, she would need counselling so that she could discuss her feelings.

The next area that was agreed to be tackled was the household cleaning. Initially it was agreed that Violet's mother would clean the house for a maximum of 30 minutes daily. Again, Violet screamed and cried, which her parents found very distressing but managed by supporting each other to resist the demands to repeat the clean.

After several weeks, Violet realised that her parents were not going to 'give in'. She agreed to accept treatment and to come to the hospital. Despite agreeing, she was extremely angry with her parents, who she believed were 'unreasonable' and that 'they ought to do what I tell them'. During her treatment, a new behaviour emerged whereby Violet would telephone her parents and demand that they tell her that 'all is OK and you won't catch an infection'. Obviously, this reassurance-seeking was not helpful in her programme. A meeting was held with the family, and it was agreed that when such requests were made, the parent would reply, 'Violet I love you very much but answering these questions is not helpful to you. I have been asked by the hospital not to answer these questions'.

After several weeks in the hospital, Violet was still insistent that she would not engage in an exposure and response prevention (ERP) programme, which she believed was 'disgusting and unreasonable'. She was still telephoning her parents both to seek reassurance and to beg them to take her home. This was an extremely difficult time for her parents as they felt guilty even though they also knew they were acting in Violet's best interests. Violet was started on a selective serotonin reuptake inhibitor, which she was happy to take, and this reduced some of her fears and worries. Still unwilling to embark on an ERP programme, a family meeting was held to discuss her future. With the support of their counsellor, Violet's parents told her that they were not willing to take her back home. Violet became very angry and abusive, and both parents were distraught. The counsellor reminded them that they were doing this for Violet's best interests. At a second meeting, Violet was calmer. Her parents explained that they would visit her and that she could come home, initially for daytime visits, but that they could no longer have her living at home. A discussion was then held as to where Violet should live. Her local social worker agreed to look for local supported accommodation.

Violet is currently settled in a hostel which is a few miles from her parents' home. Her parents visit once a week, and Violet goes home on Sunday afternoons. Her parents look more relaxed and happy. Violet is still unwilling to engage in ERP treatment but has improved in her symptoms due to the medication and also the change in environment. It is hoped she may accept ERP treatment in the future.

Violet's case is interesting because Violet herself is not keen to receive therapy. Her parents realise that for the benefit of everyone, she needs to change. It is neither ethical nor practical to 'force' Violet to accept treatment. From her point of view, she says she would be happy to remain at home and with her parents waiting on her and agreeing to her demands. This is not reasonable for her parents, who also need to live their lives. By altering what they will do in the home, Violet started to understand that life at home was changing and that she needed to think about accepting help and treatment.

Throughout the years, I have seen many people who are not willing to accept treatment with ERP at first. This can be because, at present, the treatment seems worse than the condition. Fear of the unknown is another major factor. People generally are fearful of change, and OCD can seem to be a 'reliable, good friend' rather than the life-destroying monster it appears to everyone else. It is not possible to 'do' ERP to anyone; they need to want to do it and to lead the process. The best thing to do in these cases is to leave the individual until they are ready and willing to accept treatment. This may take months, years, or even decades. Some people never decide to accept treatment. The key is to ensure they understand the treatment and to leave the door open for their return to therapy if they chose to do so.

Risk to Children When a Parent Has OCD

Children are the most vulnerable people in a family because they do not have the choices open to adults. When a parent has OCD, this can lead to a range of problems for the children. Parents who spend hours engaged in compulsive rituals may neglect their children, and occasionally in these cases, they might need to be taken into care. More frequently, there are less severe problems but still issues that need to be addressed and prevented.

Some parents with OCD incorporate their children in their compulsive rituals. This could involve extensive washing and cleaning compulsions. Indeed, I have seen children whose skin has been rubbed raw by an overzealous parent trying to 'decontaminate' them. This is unacceptable, and no child should be subjected to such treatment. If alerted to this, the children's welfare should be assessed by a qualified professional.

Parents may also demand children perform actions in a certain fashion guided by OCD, or they may restrict their children's ability to play outside or with friends and to bring friends home. Again, this is unacceptable. Children must be free to experience a 'normal' childhood, irrespective of the problems of their parents. In such situations, the children's welfare must always be the prime consideration. Again, the children need to be assessed by a qualified professional. The parent needs to stop placing these restrictions and demands on the children. This is easier said than done, but it is non-negotiable for the welfare of the children.

How Involved in Care and Treatment Should Families Be?

Assuming that the person with OCD is an adult, the level of involvement of the family and friends in the person's treatment will vary. Treatment with ERP or medication requires the person with OCD to want to engage in the treatment to try to overcome the problem. If the person with OCD wants friends and family to help with treatment, then it is best for that person to define how they can help. Similarly, the person with OCD will be able to say whether or not they would like family and friends to attend any appointments with them. It can be very difficult to see a loved one undergoing treatment and not to be asked to help, but in fact, this may be the way in which the individual is learning to take a step forward and to overcome OCD themselves. It is usually best for family and friends to ask if they can help and to leave it to the individual to decide one way or other.

Sometimes an individual with OCD is reluctant to express their fears openly, and it can take careful and sympathetic listening and support to understand the obsessions. Indeed, if there is a high degree of shame and embarrassment concerning the obsessive thoughts, they may be unwilling to discuss these with those who are closest to them. In such situations, it is important that some ground rules are still set to keep everyone in the family on 'an even keel'.

Sometimes it can be difficult for families to withhold reassurance and not provide help with compulsions because it seems as if they do not care. It is important to demonstrate care in ways which are more 'healthy' and productive. Depending on the nature of the OCD and the stage of the individual in their 'OCD journey', care may be demonstrated by going for a walk with the loved one or having family dinners and discussions on non-OCD topics.

Violence and OCD

Violence, threats, and abusive behaviour are never acceptable. Sometimes, people with OCD may 'lash out' if a relative interrupts their compulsive rituals either on purpose or accidentally. Whatever the situation, violence is always unacceptable. Family members are often reluctant to report violence to the authorities. Although this is understandable, it may not be helpful. Although violence may be 'out of character' for the individual, there is still conscious control in OCD. Ignoring and 'brushing violent episodes under the carpet' can lead to an escalation of violence. Not only is this dangerous for the person who is the victim of this violence but also it is damaging to the person with OCD. If they learn to 'lash out' whenever their compulsions are interrupted or when someone does not meet their demands, they may some day commit a very serious violent act.

The rule for those who are threatened with violence is simple: They must protect themselves. This may mean leaving the situation or contacting the police. Acting in this way is to the benefit of other family members and the person with OCD. It can be difficult because families do not wish to inflict further distress on their loved one, but it is in the best interest of everyone involved that it is crystal clear that violence of any form is unacceptable.

Key Points

- OCD is a condition which affects all family members and not just the person with OCD.
- Family members may also need help and counselling. They can ask for this through a 'carer's assessment'.

- Family members need to establish 'ground rules' about what is and what is not acceptable and what they will tolerate.

- Giving reassurance to a person with OCD offers temporary relief, but then the anxiety returns.

- Giving reassurance or taking over jobs and performing compulsions for the person with OCD makes the situation worse in the long term.

- It is difficult to stop engaging in behaviours such as reassurance-seeking or helping with compulsive rituals because it can cause extreme distress to the OCD sufferer. A frank discussion needs to be held with them before implementing the change.

- The person with OCD needs to be willing to engage in ERP; it is not a treatment that can be 'done' to them.

- People with OCD have to determine their own 'rock bottom' point and when they will accept treatment. Family members must try to ensure that their own lives are as unimpaired by their relative's OCD as possible.

- Sometimes it is necessary to make difficult decisions, such as refusing to allow a son or daughter to remain living in the house, in order to help those with OCD start to change.

- If the person with OCD is a parent, the needs of the children are paramount. Children should be free to develop, grow, explore, and form friendships free of any OCD restrictions imposed by others. If this is not the case, then the child's well-being needs to be assessed by a child health professional.

- Violence and threats are never acceptable. Family members must always protect themselves. There should be consideration about calling the police after any violence has occurred.

Chapter 10

What Can the Person with OCD Do to Help Themselves?

This final chapter will examine how someone with OCD can help themselves and seek treatment. Advice will be given on setting up a self-treatment exposure and response prevention (ERP) programme, and resources and organisations which can be helpful in achieving this are discussed. The advice will be given as a step-by-step guide for developing a personal ERP programme to tackle OCD.

This chapter will also examine what to do if an individual is having difficulty accessing help, and it will give useful contacts and organisations as well as written material.

I Have OCD But How Do I Get Help?

This section is geared towards people living in the United Kingdom but may also be applicable to other countries. OCD (and body dysmorphic disorder [BDD]) have official guidance produced by the National Institute for Health and Care Excellence (NICE). This body declares the treatment one should receive within the National Health Service (NHS) and is produced for England and Wales. In Scotland, the Scottish Intercollegiate Guidelines Network (SIGN) adopts and monitors the application of NICE guidance as well as producing some of its own guidance. In Northern Ireland, the body is NICE in Northern Ireland, which adopts and monitors the NICE guidance. The original guidance for OCD came out in 2005 but has been regularly updated. The current guidance is lengthy but can be found at www.nice.org.uk/guidance/cg31/chapter/1-Guidance. It can also be obtained from Her Majesty's Stationery Office as CG31 and is available from the following:

National Institute for Health and Clinical Excellence

MidCity Place

71 High Holborn

London, WC1V 6NA

This guidance states that everyone with OCD should have access to specialised OCD treatment. This includes psychological therapy involving ERP. The intensity of treatment offered depends on the severity of the condition, but it varies from low-intensity therapy (usually ten hours) from local psychological services in primary care to intensive specialised services funded nationally. In addition, the guidance recommends treatment with selective serotonin reuptake inhibitors (SSRIs) or clomipramine and advises that those people who do not respond to these or to ERP should additionally be offered a dopamine blocking agent (as discussed in Chapter 3).

In short, everyone in the United Kingdom should be able to receive appropriate treatment for OCD. The first thing that someone needs to do when seeking help is to visit their general practitioner (GP) and ask to be referred for psychological therapy for OCD or to be prescribed an SSRI. If there is any difficulty with this, it is worthwhile referring to the NICE Guidance CG31 (2005). All GPs should have access to psychological treatment in primary care teams (sometime known as IAPT or Increasing Access for Psychological Therapy). Many of these psychological services will also accept direct referrals from patients themselves. Every region should have such services, but the waiting lists can vary from days to months.

Once referred or receiving an appointment, most people with OCD should be offered ERP. Occasionally, other treatments may be offered if there are complicating diagnoses. For example, people with emotional instability may first need to be seen by a specialised team for treatment of this condition, or people who have experienced extreme trauma may need that addressed first. Sometimes people with OCD are offered anxiety management training. Although this can be helpful for addressing some of the symptoms of anxiety, it is not generally helpful for OCD. If a person is worried you are not receiving the correct help, then you should raise this concern with your therapist.

If the treatment in the primary care service does not help, you should be moved into secondary care services and eventually should be sent to a specialist team that specialises in OCD. Some areas of the country have specialised regional treatment centres for OCD. Unfortunately, these services are not available everywhere. In addition, there is a shortage of therapists specialising in the treatment and management of OCD. However, it is usually possible to find someone locally.

If an individual has not responded to treatment locally and has been offered the treatments mentioned previously, then they may need to be referred to a national treatment centre for OCD. For England and Wales, people who fail to respond to a range of treatments locally can be referred to a highly specialist team for OCD and BDD via the provision of NHS England Highly Specialist Services for OCD and BDD. Details can be found atwww.england.nhs.uk/wp-content/uploads/2013/06/c09-sev-ocd-boy-dysm.pdf and also at www.swlstg-tr.nhs.uk/documents/related-documents/our-services/336-national-service-referral-criteria/file. People with OCD and BDD who live in Scotland, Wales, or Northern Ireland can also be referred to these services via their health department.

What Can I Do to Help Myself?

Some people with OCD may decide to try and tackle the OCD themselves. This may be because they have a mild problem and do not wish to take time from work or other commitments that therapy may entail. Others may have tried therapy before and found that the pace was too fast and they had difficulty complying. Still others may just want to try to overcome the difficulties themselves. Whatever the reason, you should remember that overcoming OCD does involve commitment and bravery and can be difficult to do on your own. Even if you do not wish to seek professional help immediately, it may be worthwhile contacting one of the self-help groups listed later in this chapter.

Next, it is important to remember that you are not 'going mad' but have a problem with nasty, anxiety-provoking thoughts, images, or ideas. In order to cope with these thoughts, you have undoubtedly developed a number of strategies to reduce the discomfort caused by the thoughts. These strategies have been fully described in Chapter 3 and include compulsive thoughts or behaviours which reduce the anxiety, such as checking and washing compulsions as well as seeking reassurance from others or taking some precautions and avoiding situations in which the obsessional thoughts are triggered. Unfortunately, these strategies have the effect of fuelling the problem and making the situation worse. Treatment will involve stopping these behaviours and learning to face the fear without these. Some people use alcohol or drugs in an attempt to block out the anxiety. If this is the case, then it is important to first obtain help to overcome these problems before embarking on an exposure programme which is likely to initially increase anxiety levels and therefore may mean that there is a greater tendency to resort to temporary relief from drugs or alcohol.

Before embarking on a self-guided therapy programme or any therapy programme, it is wise to try to be as physically fit and healthy as possible so that you are in the best situation to tackle the programme. This means ensuring that you drink sufficient fluids, eat regular healthy meals, and try to get plenty of sleep and some exercise.

Finally, you should try to discuss options with your GP and read about the treatment options available in general and in your local area.

How Should I Set about Starting Treatment for Myself?

The first thing to do if you want to start working on your OCD is to fully assess the problem yourself. Imagine you had a magic wand and could make all your OCD symptoms go away. What would your life look like? Where would you be living? What job would you be doing? What would your social life look like?

Next, assess what you would need to do to achieve your goals. Would you need to go back to college to gain some qualifications? What would be necessary for you to learn to be more independent, etc. This list may appear daunting, but bear in mind that there is no rush, and every step in the right direction is a step nearer your goal.

It may be helpful to keep a list of your goals nearby to remind yourself of your dreams when treatment is tough. Some people place a reminder of where they are aiming next to their bed or keep it written on a card to look at when they become disheartened.

What Next?

Think about the problems and write them down. These may be similar to the following:

- 'Fear of dirt and germs for fear I may become ill and spread the infection to other people'
- 'Fear I may contract HIV'
- 'Fear I may be a paedophile and may act on this'
- 'Fear that unless I perform everything perfectly I will be rejected'
- 'Fear that unless I check doors, windows, gas, and electrical appliances, a disaster will occur'
- 'Fear that unless I perform tasks in a set way I won't feel "just right" and will be anxious and uncomfortable'

These are just a few of the possibilities. It can be difficult to identify exactly what the fear is, but it is worth spending the time to try to identify it. Many people may have more than one major fear or 'theme' of their obsessions. Identifying the fear in this way not only makes it easier to perform the next step in the ERP but also makes the OCD seem more manageable. People with OCD are often overwhelmed by their problems and feel they 'cannot see the wood for the trees'. By isolating a few 'themes' in this way, it can make you realise that the problem is, indeed, containable.

How Do I Develop My Goals of Treatment?

After you have identified the fear(s), consider what task you would be able to do to demonstrate to yourself and others that you have overcome it. For example, for a fear of contamination, the task might be 'Visit a public toilet, sit on the toilet seat without using disinfectant, use the toilet and leave with a 30-second hand wash'. For fear of paedophilia, it might be 'Sit in a place full of children without checking'. For fear of disaster occurring in the house, it might be 'Leave the house without checking'. For perfectionistic fears, it might be 'Deliberately leave the house without checking my hair and clothes'.

Although this stage is not essential, it can help with devising the hierarchy.

Set out a 'Ladder' or 'Hierarchy' of Fears

In this step, the stages on the way to facing the fear are identified *without performing any anxiety-reducing compulsive rituals or reassurance-seeking*. It is important to remember that these tasks need to be performed without the compulsions, and the anxiety needs to be scored in this way. For some compulsions, such as 'hand washing', there will still be a ban on the compulsions and a whole 'new' way of hand washing will be introduced. Once you have identified the stages in this way, score the anxiety/discomfort you think you will feel whilst engaging in them. A useful scoring system is to score as follows:

0 = no anxiety

2 = mild anxiety

4 = moderate anxiety

6 = severe anxiety

8 = extreme anxiety/cannot be higher/panic

As an example, Table 10.1 presents a hierarchy of someone who has fear of dirt and germs for fear of contracting and spreading an illness.

The hierarchy may contain many more items than listed in Table 10.1. It is also important to remember that the exposure tasks should be performed *without performing compulsive rituals*. With regard to hand washing, clearly everyone needs to wash their hands during the day, but the key here is the extent and way in which this is done. Most people with 'decontamination rituals' perform them in set ways. For example, they may always wash in running water and may wash beyond their wrists. The hand wash may take several minutes. In the exposure programme, all hand washing except that before meals or food preparation should be banned. Hand washing should involve putting some water in the basin and then washing to the wrist only for approximately 30 seconds (or the time it takes to sing 'Happy Birthday to You' in your head). Programmes should not be performed immediately before preparing meals but, rather, are best performed after eating, and after the hand washing has been performed, to prolong exposure time.

Table 10.1 Hierarchy for someone who has fear of dirt and germs for fear of contracting and spreading an illness

Task (to be performed without washing rituals)	Anxiety rating (0–8)
Touch door handles in home (apart from toilet handles)	1
Get dressed without hand washing in between	2
Touch toilet door handles in home	3
Touch shop door handles, pedestrian crossing buttons	4
Bring items home from supermarket without washing outside packaging	5
Prepare food without first washing hands repeatedly	6
Touch public toilet door handle	8
Use public toilet	8

How Should I Perform My Exposure Tasks?

Exposure tasks need to be performed consistently and regularly. You need to start at the bottom of the hierarchy and not jump to higher levels. Stick with one or two items and conquer those before moving on.

The exposure must also be performed regularly, ideally three times a day but at least daily if you are to experience benefit. Record your anxiety during each exposure task (using the same 0–8 scale discussed previously). You will find that initially your anxiety will last for two or three hours, but the more you practice, the shorter the anxiety will last, and the level of anxiety will also decline.

You may find yourself performing compulsive rituals before you realise it. This is normal and natural. If you do perform the compulsions, then go back and re-expose yourself to the fear. With decontamination compulsions, after touching the item it can be useful to touch your body, clothes, and hair and, if possible, lick your hands because this is much more difficult to 'undo'.

Compulsive thoughts are much more difficult to control. For this reason, it is often best to make a recording of the obsessive fear-provoking thought and listen to this on repeat mode on your mobile phone or similar portable device whilst performing exposure. It is difficult to always 'undo' the exposure if the exposure is repeated.

Some people try to 'jump around' the hierarchy and suddenly perform a much more difficult item. This is not a good idea. People who do this end up disappointed and disillusioned. Remember that you need to learn to walk before you can run. It takes time, but the gradual approach is best.

Once the items at the bottom of your hierarchy are causing little or no anxiety, it is time to step up to the items causing moderate anxiety. You will probably find that having done the groundwork with easier items, these more difficult items are now easier than you expected and may only cause mild anxiety. Once you have conquered the items causing moderate anxiety, move on to the more difficult items.

At the end when you have performed all the items on the programme, take stock of where you are with respect to the initially stated therapy goals. Think about your life goals and whether now is the time to move forward by taking on a training course or other challenge. Remember that obsessions can expand to fill a vacuum in your life and so keeping busy can be useful in the battle to overcome OCD.

Troubleshooting

Therapy does not always work out as it does in books. There are certain things you need to be aware of.

First, the obsessions will still persist for a long time even after you have faced up to them. The important thing is not to give in to the compulsions. Eventually, over time, the obsessions will fade.

In addition, sometimes as you start to tackle one obsession, another even worse obsession develops. Do not get distracted by this. Remind yourself that, however unpleasant, it is just an obsession, and once you have dealt with the one obsession, you can move on to dealing with the next one. Do not get disheartened – this is all normal and will just take time. Remember, you will overcome the problems in the end.

What If the Anxiety Is Not Coming Down?

Have you exposed yourself for long enough without performing compulsions? Remember it will often take two or three hours before the anxiety comes down. The other issue is whether you have performed the exposure three times a day. Although it does not have to always be three times a day, it must be at least once or twice a day if you are to achieve good results. Three times a day usually leads to the quickest results. Have you been honest about your compulsions? Are you still getting some reassurance or performing other compulsions which will serve to maintain your anxiety? However tempting it can be to engage in compulsions, they really do help maintain anxiety.

If you are sure you have dealt with all the previously mentioned issues, then it may be worthwhile to consider either trying a course of SSRIs or trying some professional help.

Reward and Praise Yourself

Finally, remember that ERP is far from easy. You need to be very brave to face your fears. Once you have truly faced your fears, you need to reward yourself. Take stock and pride in what you have achieved. Remember that true heroes experience anxiety but face it. That is what you have been doing, so you deserve to be kind to yourself. OCD is not a weakness nor a character flaw but, rather, a very real illness, just as any physical illness is not a character flaw or weakness. Praise yourself for what you are doing for yourself, and remind yourself of where you are heading. Do not get disheartened if progress seems slow; it is much better to have a slow but effective programme than a 'miracle cure' which collapses within a short time.

Set yourself small rewards after completing your programmes – whatever you enjoy that does not completely break the bank. Maybe a relaxing soak in a bath (assuming you do not have washing compulsions!). Perhaps a walk in the park or a favourite meal? Pamper yourself a little!

Good luck and remember that even people who do not succeed the first time often succeed when they try again. Be kind to yourself, and keep your sense of humour!

Are There Any Organisations That Offer Help and Support?

There are a variety of self-help and support organisations for people with OCD and their families. Many counties have several organisations; Table 10.2 is geared to the United Kingdom.

Table 10.2 Organisations in the United Kingdom that help people with OCD

Organisation	Website	What they offer	Notes
OCD Action	www.ocdaction.org.uk	Helpline; website containing information on OCD; books available online; local support; conferences for people with OCD and their families; lobby government and others about OCD matters	It is the United Kingdom's largest OCD charity.
OCD UK	http://ocduk.org	Helpline; website containing information on OCD; books available online; local support; conferences for people with OCD and their families; lobby government and others about OCD matters	
TOP UK (Triumph Over Phobia and OCD)	www.topuk.org	Offers local treatment groups in some areas; website containing information; lobbying of government and others about issues pertaining to OCD and phobic disorders	It offers its own treatment groups for those with mild to moderate OCD or who do not wish to go through the NHS.
MIND	www.mind.org.uk	Mental health charity which provides information on a variety of mental health issues; lobbying of government and others on mental health issues	MIND media awards are prestigious awards awarded for informative and sensitive portrayal or information on mental health issues.
International OCD Foundation	https://iocdf.org	Website containing information for people with OCD and health care professionals; training courses available for professionals	This has arisen from the US-based OCD Foundation, which seeks to inform the public, educate professionals, and raise awareness of OCD.

Key Points

- There are various ways in which you can access therapy. In the United Kingdom, all areas should have access to psychological therapies in primary care.

- In the United Kingdom, the National Institute for Care and Health Care Excellence has published guidance on the treatments people with OCD and body dysmorphic disorder should receive. These are published in England but accepted in other areas of the United Kingdom.

- Self-help means first identifying and setting out the problem and trying to think of what your life would be like without OCD.

- A hierarchy of fears should be constructed of exposure tasks which would cause anxiety when performed without compulsions.

- Exposure tasks should start with easier ones which should be performed ideally three times a day.

- Initially, anxiety will take two or three hours to subside completely.

- Once easier tasks have been achieved with ease, move on to slightly more difficult items.

- Do not jump to the most difficult items; take it slow.

- Be kind to yourself; ERP is difficult and you need to recognise your achievements. OCD is not evidence of weakness or a character flaw but, rather, a very real illness.

- If the treatment does not seem to be working after at least a week of trying exposure to one or two items, think about whether you are performing the tasks often enough, for long enough, and without compulsive rituals.

- If, despite performing ERP correctly, you do not improve, it is worthwhile thinking about medication or psychological help.

- Reward yourself and take pride in your efforts. ERP is very difficult and you need to be brave to tackle it.

- You are not alone, and there are many organisations and self-help groups that can help you.

Glossary

Aripiprazole: This is a medication which acts to block dopamine in the brain and can be a helpful addition to treatment with the serotonin reuptake inhibitors (SRIs) for some people. Aripiprazole tends to have fewer side effects than some of the older drugs and is less likely to cause drowsiness.

Asperger's syndrome: See *autism*. A development condition which is part of the autistic disorders. This condition varies in severity from mild to severe. In general, people with Asperger's syndrome may have difficulty understanding other people and their motives and may also have difficulty interpreting other people's body language. Some people with Asperger's syndrome may develop repetitive behaviours which resemble OCD, and some will develop true OCD.

Atypical dopamine blockers: Dopamine blockers are drugs which can be used to increase the efficacy of the SRIs in some people with OCD. Atypical dopamine blockers are a group of newer drugs which act on dopamine and were introduced after 1990. They tend to have fewer side effects compared to the older dopamine blockers.

Autism (autistic spectrum disorder): This is a lifelong developmental disorder (i.e., it starts in infancy). People with autism may be extremely clever, but they have difficulty understanding other people's body language and motives and consequently have difficulty in social situations. Some people with autistic spectrum disorders may develop repetitive behaviours which resemble OCD, and some will develop true OCD. Approximately 1 in 100 people have autism, and it is more common in men than in women.

Autoimmune: The body has many specialised protective cells which are designed to fight infection and keep people healthy. In autoimmune disorders, the process has gone wrong, and these protective cells can start to attack parts of the body they are designed to keep safe. Examples of autoimmune disorder include rheumatoid arthritis, in which the joints are attacked; Type 1 (or childhood-onset) diabetes, in which the pancreas is attacked; and coeliac disease, in which the gut becomes abnormal and develops a reaction to gluten (a component of wheat).

Behaviour therapy: This is a practical form of therapy with the basic belief that many psychological symptoms are a result of behaviours which make the situation worse. As these behaviours are learned, the individual can learn to replace them with more helpful behaviours. For example, if a person has a horrible, intrusive OCD thought, the compulsive behaviour serves to fuel the obsessive thought and make it more frequent and severe. Learning to resist the compulsive behaviour results in reduced anxiety and discomfort.

Body dysmorphic disorder (BDD): This is a condition which is similar to OCD in many ways. The individual, however, is preoccupied by a perceived defect in their appearance and thoughts of which preoccupy them throughout the day. These thoughts often lead to checking behaviours, including spending excessive amounts of time looking in mirrors. There is also frequent avoidance, and some people may totally avoid looking at themselves in the mirror and may only go out whilst concealed by wearing makeup or in darkness or, indeed, may avoid leaving the house entirely.

Capsulotomy: A form of brain surgery very rarely used to try to control the symptoms of OCD which have not responded to other methods. Extremely rarely used in the United Kingdom.

Cingulotomy: A form of brain surgery very rarely used to try to control the symptoms of OCD which have not responded to other methods. Extremely rarely used.

Citalopram: A modern antidepressant drug which has a direct effect on the symptoms of OCD irrespective of whether the person is depressed or not. It works by reducing the reuptake of serotonin, a neurotransmitter which appears to be low in certain areas of the brain in people with OCD.

Clomipramine: An older type of antidepressant which was found in the 1980s to have a direct effect on obsessive compulsive symptoms. It was discovered that this anti-obsessive effect was mainly due to its effect of increasing serotonin in certain parts of the brain and appeared separate from its antidepressant action. Although a very useful drug, it tends to have more side effects than the more modern selective serotonin reuptake inhibitors (SSRIs).

Clozapine: An atypical dopamine blocking drug. This is often used in people with schizophrenia who do not respond to first-line therapy. There is evidence that it can precipitate OCD symptoms in some people.

Cognitive behaviour therapy (CBT): A practical form of therapy used for a variety of mental health conditions. In this therapy, the emphasis is on the 'here and now' rather than looking at the past. It involves either examining thoughts and also carrying out real-life exercises to test out these beliefs or helping people overcome their fears by facing them in a structured way.

Cognitive therapy: See *cognitive behaviour therapy*. This refers to the process of examining a person's thoughts and beliefs and encouraging the individual to challenge those that are unhelpful to them.

Compulsion: A thought or action which is designed to reduce or prevent the effect of an obsessive thought. However, either the compulsion is not in reality associated with the obsessive thought or it is clearly excessive. Compulsions tend to fuel obsessive thoughts and make them more frequent and more persistent. Examples include cleaning obsessions for people with fear of contamination by dirt or germs.

Covert compulsions: This refers to compulsions which are carried out in an individual's head and are not obvious behaviours. An example is someone who fears they may cause harm to others by 'lashing out' at them. After they have passed other people, they may feel the urge to imagine every movement they made to ensure they did not harm anyone. After they have done this, they will often doubt their memory and repeat the thought until their memory is muddled by repeating it so often.

Deep brain stimulation (DBS): A recently introduced potential treatment for the most profound forms of OCD that do not respond to conventional treatments. This involves inserting small electrodes into the brain and, using electrical impulses, stimulating specific areas of the brain to reduce and prevent obsessions and compulsions. It does not cause brain damage and has therefore been thought of as 'reversible brain surgery'. It does, however, involve major surgery.

Dermatillomania: See *skin picking disorder*.

Dopamine blocking drugs: These are drugs which act to block the action of dopamine. In larger doses, they can be used as antipsychotic drugs, but in OCD they are used in lower doses to enhance the effect of the SRI drugs. The older drugs are known as 'typical' and tend to have more side effects than the newer 'atypical' or 'second-generation' drugs.

Escitalopram: A modern antidepressant drug which has a direct effect on the symptoms of OCD irrespective of whether the person is depressed or not. It works by reducing the reuptake of serotonin, a neurotransmitter which appears to be low in certain areas of the brain in people with OCD.

Exposure and response prevention (ERP): Treatment for OCD which involves working through a structured programme of prolonged graded exposure or, in other words, facing the anxiety- or discomfort-inducing situations for sufficient time to allow the anxiety/discomfort to subside without performing compulsive rituals.

Fluoxetine: A modern antidepressant drug which has a direct effect on the symptoms of OCD irrespective of whether the person is depressed or not. It works by reducing the reuptake of serotonin, a neurotransmitter which appears to be low in certain areas of the brain in people with OCD.

Fluvoxamine: A modern antidepressant drug which has a direct effect on the symptoms of OCD irrespective of whether the person is depressed or not. It works by reducing the reuptake of serotonin, a neurotransmitter which appears to be low in certain areas of the brain in people with OCD.

Frontal lobotomy: See *lobotomy*.

Glial cell: A type of cell found in the brain which seems to modulate or exercise some control over the neurotransmitters.

Glutamate: A neurotransmitter which has multiple effects on the neurones. It is in the brain in large concentrations, but too little or too much glutamate is not beneficial to brain functioning and health.

Haloperidol: Atypical dopamine blocker.

Health anxiety: An anxiety disorder which has many similarities to OCD. In this case, the distressing thoughts concern specific or general health issues. Once the individual has anxious thoughts about their health, they normally check in a ritualistic way. For example, some people may repeatedly check their bodies for lumps which they worry about. They may also seek repeated reassurance from friends or relatives or repeatedly visit their general practitioner or hospitals for reassurance and to ask for more and repeated physical tests.

Hierarchy: A list or ladder of situations placed in order of increasing anxiety/discomfort.

Hoarding disorder: A disorder in which an individual collects large numbers of items beyond reasonable amounts. Individuals generally have difficulty in that they cannot resist collecting large amounts of objects and they have extreme difficulty disposing of items. Hoarding can be extremely serious, leading to social impairments as well as risk to health via inability to clean around the hoard, fire risk of a large number of items, and the risk that the individual may be crushed by the falling of a large number of objects.

Limbic leucotomy: A form of brain surgery very rarely used to try to control the symptoms of OCD which have not responded to other methods. Extremely rarely used.

Lobotomy: An early form of brain surgery performed in the 1940s and early 1950s to try to alleviate a number of the symptoms in severe psychiatric illnesses. The development and use of powerful antipsychotic drugs in the mid-1950s rendered this procedure obsolete. Occasionally, this had been used for very profound OCD.

National Institute for Health and Care Excellence (NICE): This body provides national guidance and advice to improve health and social care in the United Kingdom.

Neurones: These are nerve cells which transmit messages to each other throughout the brain.

Obsession: An obsession is a thought, image, or impulse which intrudes on an individual's consciousness and is anxiety-provoking and/or distressing. These thoughts are usually totally out of character with the individual. For example, a law-abiding and caring man may have thoughts about molesting children; these thoughts are totally abhorrent to him. A devoted mother may have thoughts of violently attacking her children; these thoughts distress her greatly. A religious person may have blasphemous thoughts which can cause extreme distress. Some people have worries about 'contamination' and spreading of dirt or germs, and others worry that something bad may happen unless they are very careful in everyday life. Common obsessions include the following:

- Fear of contamination causing harm to self or others
- Fear of harm occurring by the individual failing to perform a vital action (e.g., switching off gas taps)
- Fear of harm occurring by performing an act of violence or similar
- Religious obsessions
- Fear of loss of objects or information

Obsessive compulsive and related disorders: These are a group of disorders which are thought to be related and include the following:

- OCD
- Body dysmorphic disorder
- Hoarding disorder
- Hair pulling disorder (trichotillomania)
- Skin picking disorder
- OCD resulting from another cause, such as brain damage, infection, or substance misuse

These disorders are sometimes also referred to as obsessive compulsive spectrum disorders.

Obsessive compulsive spectrum disorders: See *obsessive compulsive and related disorders*. In addition to the group of disorders categorised as obsessive compulsive and related disorders, other conditions including health anxiety as well as eating disorders and pathological gambling are included under this term. In general, it refers to any condition in which there are difficulties in compulsive behaviours, impulsive behaviours, or both.

Olanzepine: This is one of the newer or 'atypical' dopamine blocking drugs. Although used in people with psychotic illnesses in higher dosages, it is sometimes useful as an addition to an SRI in low doses for people with OCD.

Overt compulsions: These are compulsions which can be seen – for example, someone with extensive washing compulsions or someone who checks door locks or light switches by repeatedly touching, pulling, or switching them.

Oxytocin: This is a chemical produced in the hypothalamus area of the brain and released by the pituitary. It has a role in social-bonding, sexual reproduction, and also childbirth and lactation. It is sometimes referred to as the 'love hormone'.

Paediatric autoimmune neurological syndrome: This is a controversial idea and refers to an identical picture as paediatric autoimmune neuropsychiatric disorders associated with streptococcal infection (PANDAS), but it is suggested that other common bacterial infections (or occasionally viral infections) may also result in OCD in susceptible children, which starts suddenly and is sometimes accompanied by dramatic movement disorders.

Paediatric autoimmune neuropsychiatric disorders associated with streptococcal infection (PANDAS): This represents a controversial idea that some rapid-onset OCD symptoms which can occur in childhood may be accompanied by other neurological symptoms such as an inability to control movements of the limbs or trunk or an inability to stand up and walk without falling. This condition is thought to occur in susceptible individuals following an illness such as a sore throat. Bacterial sore throats (which are less common than those caused by viruses) can occasionally be caused by bacteria known as streptococci. These infections are common in childhood, whereas PANDAS is rare.

Paroxetine: A modern antidepressant drug which has a direct effect on the symptoms of OCD irrespective of whether the person is depressed or not. It works by reducing the reuptake of serotonin, a neurotransmitter which appears to be low in certain areas of the brain in people with OCD.

Personality disorder: This refers to a condition whereby the individual differs in many ways from an average person in how they think, view the world, experience emotions, or relate to others. There are many different types of personality disorder. Some examples are given here. People with obsessive personality disorder tend to be scrupulous, punctual, and rather pedantic individuals who strive for perfection and may become 'workaholics'. They tend to differ from people with OCD because they do not believe these traits interfere with their lives but tend to blame others for not being perfect. People with emotional unstable personality disorder have extreme difficulty dealing with and handling emotions and may use self-destructive behaviours as a result. These unhelpful behaviours may include self-harm, abuse of alcohol or drugs, and binge eating.

Prefrontal lobotomy: See *lobotomy*.

Selective serotonin reuptake inhibitors (SSRIs): These are drugs which act on the serotonin system of the brain. SSRIs are known to be helpful in reducing the symptoms of OCD and tend to have fewer and less severe side effects compared to the older serotonin reuptake inhibiting drug clomipramine. SSRIs comprise the following:

- Sertraline
- Fluoxetine
- Paroxetine
- Fluvoxamine
- Citalopram
- Escitalopram

Serotonin: This is a chemical found in the brain as well as other parts of the body. In the brain, it acts as a neurotransmitter and thus helps in the passage of information along the brain cells.

Serotonin reuptake inhibitors (SRIs): These are drugs which are known to be helpful in reducing the symptoms of OCD. They act by increasing the levels of the neurotransmitter serotonin in specific areas of the brain by preventing it from being absorbed quickly back into the nerve cells. SRIs comprise the older antidepressant drug clomipramine and the newer SSRI drugs.

Sertraline: A modern antidepressant drug which has a direct effect on the

symptoms of OCD irrespective of whether the person is depressed or not. It works by reducing the reuptake of serotonin, a neurotransmitter which appears to be low in certain areas of the brain in people with OCD.

Skin picking disorder (dermatillomania): This is a condition in which the individual feels the urge to pick the skin to the point that they usually have visible wounds. The most common areas affected are the face and lips, but it can involve any part of the body. As with hair pulling disorder, it is most common in teenagers and young adults, and it is more common in women than men. It is included as one of the obsessive compulsive and related conditions.

Strep sore throat: This is a bacterial throat infection in which the throat and tonsils are red and sore. It is caused by bacteria known as streptococci. Approximately 15–40 per cent of throat infections in children are caused by streptococci; far fewer throat infections in adults are caused by streptococci. It can be treated with antibiotics. Some people believe that a tiny number of children with this infection may rarely develop PANDAS after the infection.

Subcaudate tractotomy: A form of brain surgery very rarely used to try to control the symptoms of OCD which have not responded to other methods. Extremely rarely used.

Tics: These are involuntary movements of which the individual is aware they are doing but which they feel unable to stop performing. Tics frequently involve the muscles of the face and can include grimacing or blinking repeatedly; such movements of the muscles are known as motor tics. Also, people with tics frequently utter involuntary sounds, such as repetitive throat clearing. Sometimes motor tics can involve muscles which would not be visible to others, such as clenching of abdominal muscles. Tics of both types are common in childhood and may disappear spontaneously without the need for any treatment.

Tourette's syndrome: This condition affects approximately 1 in 100 children and can often disappear spontaneously as they grow but can also come and go throughout childhood. It consists of muscular tics as well as vocal tics. Tourette's syndrome is not dangerous, and many children and adults do not require treatment. The most profound and dramatic version in which the individual utters obscenities is very rare, occurring in fewer than one in ten people with Tourette's syndrome. Up to half of individuals with Tourette's syndrome have some OCD symptoms, and approximately 1 in 3 of these individuals will have clinical OCD.

Transcranial magnetic stimulation (TMS): This is an experimental treatment in usage for OCD. It involves applying strong magnets outside the head in an attempt to 'dampen' down certain areas of the brain on a temporary basis. The magnetic fields are produced by using electric currents, and the resulting magnetism can be pinpointed to specific areas of the brain. It has been shown to be useful for major depression and also certain types of pain. Currently, there is insufficient evidence to fully recommend it for the treatment of OCD.

Trichotillomania (hair pulling disorder): This is a condition whereby the individual feels compelled to pull out their hair. This is frequently on the head but can involve other hair, such as eyebrows or eyelashes. The individual will often describe the buildup of tension and then relief when the hair is plucked. However, it often results in guilt and remorse. Many people with hair pulling disorders end up with bald patches. This condition is most common amongst teenagers and young adults, and it is more common in young women than in men.

Resources

Information Sources

General introduction to OCD and its treatment

National Health Service (NHS) choices (United Kingdom)
www.nhs.uk/conditions/Obsessive-compulsive-disorder/Pages/Introduction.aspx#treatment

Royal College of Psychiatrists (United Kingdom)
www.rcpsych.ac.uk/healthadvice/problemsdisorders/obsessivecompulsivedisorder.aspx

National Institute for Mental Health (United States)
www.nimh.nih.gov/health/topics/obsessive-compulsive-disorder-ocd/index.shtml

Description of treatment from the Australian Psychological Society
www.psychology.org.au/for-the-public/Psychology-topics/Obsessive-compulsive-disorder

Information from the National Institute for Health and Clinical Excellence (NICE)

A full description of the treatments that can be expected within the NHS is given at
www.nice.org.uk/guidance/cg31/chapter/1-Guidance

or it can be obtained from Her Majesty's Stationery Office as CG31 and is available from

National Institute for Health and Clinical Excellence
MidCity Place
71 High Holborn
London, WC1V 6NA

Description of services available in the United Kingdom

Specialist services in England
www.england.nhs.uk/wp-content/uploads/2013/06/c09-sev-ocd-boy-dysm.pdf

Specialist services available throughout the United Kingdom
www.swlstg-tr.nhs.uk/documents/related-documents/our-services/336-national-service-referral-criteria/file

Consensus statement from the British Association for Psychopharmacology

A description of the various drugs used in anxiety disorders and obsessive compulsive disorder
www.bap.org.uk/pdfs/BAP_Guidelines-Anxiety.pdf

Self-Help Organisations

OCD Action: A UK-based organisation providing support as well as information and meetings for people living with OCD and their relatives, friends, and carers.
www.ocdaction.org.uk

OCD-UK: A UK-based organisation providing support as well as information and meetings for people living with OCD and their relatives, friends, and carers.
www.ocduk.org

TOP UK: A UK-based organisation offering support and treatment groups for people with phobic anxiety and OCD.
www.topuk.org

International OCD Foundation: A
US-based organisation offering
conferences and information
for people with OCD and also
professionals.
https://iocdf.org

SANE: An Australian-based charity for
mental health offering information and
fora for conditions including OCD.
www.sane.org/mental-health-
and-illness/facts-and-guides/
obsessive-compulsive-disorder

Other Organisations

International College for Obsessive-
Compulsive Spectrum Disorders
(ICOCS): An international
organisation which sets out to
promote research in OCD and
related disorders and to produce
public statements to improve OCD
treatment internationally.
www.icocs.org

International OCD Foundation: A
US-based organisation aiming to
promote awareness about OCD,
promote research in OCD, and
provide information to professionals
and people with OCD.
https://iocdf.org

Further Reading

Autobiographical books written by people who have experienced OCD

*The Man Who Couldn't Stop: The Truth
about OCD* by David Adam. London:
Picador, 2015.
An autobiographical book written by a
journalist which tells of his journey
through treatment for OCD.

*The Walking Worried: 'A Young Man's
Journey with OCD'* by Aron Bennett.
Brentwood, UK: Chipmunka
Publishing, 2015.

An autobiographical book written by
a young man who was studying
law and who eventually received
appropriate treatment for his
OCD.

Self-Help Books Written by Professionals

*Mindfulness Workbook for OCD:
A Guide to Overcoming Obsessions
and Compulsions Using Mindfulness
and Cognitive Behaviour Therapy*
by Jon Hershfield and Tom Corboy.
New York, NY: New Harbinger,
2014.
This book concentrates on the specific
approach to OCD using mainly
mindfulness and CBT. It does
not examine other aspects of
treatment.

*Break Free from OCD: Overcoming
Obsessive Compulsive Disorder
with CBT* by Fiona Challacombe,
Victoria Bream Oldfield, and Paul M.
Salkovskis. Chatham, UK: Vermilion,
2011.
This book focusses on the CBT
approach to OCD. It does not
explore psychopharmacological
or other NICE-approved
approaches.

*Obsessive Compulsive Disorder – The
Essential Guide* by Joanna Jast.
Peterborough, UK: Need2Know,
2011.
This is a more general book which
examines what constitutes OCD
and takes a broader approach
to treatment. It offers a concise
overview in 120 pages.

*The OCD Workbook: Your Guide to
Breaking Free from Obsessive–
Compulsive Disorder*, 3rd edition,
by Bruce M. Hyman. New York, NY:
New Harbinger, 2010.
Another book purely focussing on
CBT approaches to OCD.

Overcoming Obsessive Thoughts: How to Gain Control of Your OCD by Christine Purdon. New York, NY: New Harbinger, 2010.

Another book purely focussing on CBT approaches to OCD.

Overcoming Obsessive Compulsive Disorder by David Veale and Rob Willson. London: Constable & Robinson, 2005.

Another book purely focussing on CBT approaches to OCD.

Breaking Free from OCD: A CBT Guide for Young People and Their Families by Jo Derisley. London: Kingsley, 2008.

A CBT self-help guide for children and young people.

What to Do When Your Brain Gets Stuck: A Kid's Guide to Overcoming OCD by Dawn Huebner and Bonnie Matthews. Washington, DC: Margination Press, 2007.

A CBT self-help guide for children and young people.

Multi-author Books Written by Professionals and for Professionals

Clinical Guide to Obsessive–Compulsive and Related Disorders by Jon E. Grant, Samuel R. Chamberlain, and Brian L. Odlaug. New York, NY: Oxford University Press, 2014.

This book has is comprehensive and eclectic. However, it briefly mentions treatments and does not have any depth in any of the disorders. It is predominantly written for professionals and thus is a useful aide-memoire for this group.

Obsessive Compulsive Disorder: Current Science and Clinical Practice edited by Joshi Zohar. Bognor Regis, UK: Wiley, 2012.

Written for a professional audience, this multi-author book comprehensively covers the theories of OCD, its development and maintenance, and its treatment.

Handbook on Obsessive–Compulsive and Related Disorders edited by Katharine A. Phillips and Dan J. Stein. Washington, DC: American Psychiatric Association, 2015.

This is a multi-author book written for professionals that describes various subtypes of the obsessive compulsive and related disorders based on the DSM-5 classification. There are separate chapters on OCD and on trichotillomania, body dysmorphic disorder, tic disorders, and so on.

Index